DMSO Bible

The Ultimate Guide to Healing, Pain Relief, and Natural Treatments with Dimethyl Sulfoxide

Dr. Maxwell G. C. Philip

TABLE OF CONTENTS

Introduction

In the journey toward holistic health and natural remedies, Dimethyl Sulfoxide, commonly known as DMSO, stands out as one of the most versatile and impactful substances in the field. This book, *DMSO Bible: The Ultimate Guide to Healing, Pain Relief, and Natural Treatments with Dimethyl Sulfoxide*, aims to bring clarity to the science, applications, and benefits of DMSO, guiding you through its various uses and best practices for a safe, effective experience. DMSO may be unfamiliar to some and surrounded by misconceptions for others, but by diving into this book, you're taking the first step to understanding this powerful healing agent and how it can transform your approach to pain relief, inflammation management, and overall well-being.

What is DMSO?

DMSO, or Dimethyl Sulfoxide, is a sulphur-based organic compound derived from lignin, a substance found in the cell walls of plants. First synthesised as a byproduct of paper manufacturing, DMSO quickly caught the interest of scientists and medical professionals for its unique properties and applications. Chemically, DMSO is known as a "polar aprotic solvent," which means it can dissolve both polar and nonpolar compounds and penetrate biological membranes easily. These properties allow DMSO to act as a carrier, delivering other substances deep into tissues and cells, which enhances the effectiveness of treatments and supports healing on a cellular level.

One of DMSO's most remarkable qualities is its ability to permeate skin and cell membranes without causing harm. This characteristic allows it to act as a carrier agent, making it valuable in medical applications for delivering other compounds directly to areas of injury or pain. It is also an antioxidant, anti-inflammatory, and pain reliever, making it highly versatile and beneficial for various health conditions.

Since its discovery in the late 19th century and subsequent development in the 20th century, DMSO has been widely studied for its potential in medical and alternative health fields. While it has been approved for certain medical uses—such as treating interstitial cystitis in the United States—its broad-spectrum benefits remain largely underutilised and underappreciated.

Why Choose DMSO for Healing?

DMSO is a powerful natural remedy that addresses many common health concerns without the need for synthetic chemicals or invasive treatments. Unlike conventional medications that may come with a range of side effects, DMSO offers a natural alternative that works with the body's processes to relieve pain, reduce inflammation, and promote healing. Here are a few key reasons why DMSO has become a go-to solution for those seeking a more holistic approach to health:

1. **Broad Application**: DMSO is effective for numerous conditions, from chronic joint pain to skin wounds, nerve pain, and respiratory issues. This versatility means it can serve as a "one-stop shop" for many ailments, eliminating the need for multiple medications.

2. **Non-Toxic and Gentle**: DMSO, derived from natural sources, is generally well-tolerated by the body. When used correctly, it has fewer side effects than many traditional painkillers or anti-inflammatory medications, making it a safer choice for long-term use.

3. **Penetrating Power**: Unlike most topical treatments that work only on the surface, DMSO penetrates deeply, delivering relief to underlying tissues and providing a more lasting effect. This quality also allows DMSO to enhance the effectiveness of

other natural remedies, as it can "carry" them deeper into the body.

4. **Anti-Inflammatory and Antioxidant Benefits**: DMSO helps reduce inflammation, which is a common cause of pain and many chronic diseases. It also fights oxidative stress, neutralising free radicals and preventing cellular damage, which can accelerate ageing and the development of various conditions.

5. **Natural Pain Relief**: Many people turn to DMSO for its pain-relieving effects, which can alleviate conditions such as arthritis, back pain, headaches, and muscle aches. It's a natural analgesic, making it a healthier alternative to over-the-counter pain medications that may have adverse side effects.

In an age where people are increasingly sceptical of synthetic drugs and eager for natural alternatives, DMSO offers an effective solution grounded in both nature and science. Its ability to treat such a broad spectrum of ailments makes it a valuable addition to any holistic health regimen.

Overview of DMSO's Health Benefits

DMSO's health benefits are extensive, making it one of the most versatile natural remedies available. Here's an overview of its main health benefits:

- **Pain Relief**: As an analgesic, DMSO helps to alleviate pain almost instantly, making it a favourite for individuals suffering from chronic pain conditions such as arthritis, sports injuries, and back pain. It's especially effective because it penetrates deep into tissues and can provide longer-lasting relief than surface-level treatments.
- **Anti-Inflammatory Action**: DMSO reduces inflammation by suppressing the body's inflammatory responses at the cellular level. This is particularly

beneficial for conditions such as rheumatoid arthritis, tendonitis, and other inflammatory disorders.

- **Skin Healing**: For burns, cuts, bruises, and other skin injuries, DMSO promotes faster healing and reduces the risk of infection. It also minimises the formation of scar tissue by encouraging proper collagen alignment.

- **Improved Circulation**: DMSO supports better blood flow and circulation, which can be helpful for people with circulation issues or conditions that benefit from improved blood flow, such as diabetic neuropathy or varicose veins.

- **Antimicrobial and Antifungal Properties**: DMSO has natural antimicrobial properties that can help fight off bacteria, viruses, and fungi, making it effective for treating certain infections and skin conditions.

- **Nerve Regeneration**: DMSO has shown promise in supporting nerve repair and relieving nerve pain, making it beneficial for people with conditions like neuropathy or other nerve-related issues.

- **Respiratory Benefits**: DMSO can act as a mucolytic agent, helping to thin mucus and relieve respiratory conditions like bronchitis, asthma, and chronic obstructive pulmonary disease (COPD).
- **Antioxidant Power**: As an antioxidant, DMSO neutralises free radicals that cause cellular damage. This quality makes it useful in slowing down degenerative processes and promoting overall cellular health.

Addressing Common Misconceptions and Myths

Despite its proven benefits and decades of research, DMSO remains controversial and misunderstood. Several myths and misconceptions persist, often due to a lack of awareness and resistance from the mainstream medical community. Here are a few of the most common misunderstandings about DMSO:

1. **Myth: DMSO is Unsafe for Human Use**
   While it's true that DMSO can be harmful if used incorrectly or in overly high doses, when used properly and following safety guidelines, it is safe and effective. In fact, DMSO has FDA approval for treating certain conditions, and there is a wealth of scientific literature attesting to its safety profile.

2. **Myth: DMSO is Only for Veterinary Use**
   DMSO is often used in veterinary medicine, especially for treating horses with joint pain and inflammation. However, it is also effective for humans and has been used successfully for decades in clinical and at-home applications. Its use in animals doesn't negate its benefits for people but rather speaks to its versatility and effectiveness across species.

3. **Myth: DMSO Has No Scientific Basis**
   This misconception stems from a lack of awareness of the studies and clinical trials that support DMSO's use. Research has shown DMSO's efficacy in pain relief, inflammation reduction, and more. Scientific studies are readily available to demonstrate the compound's pharmacological benefits, mechanisms, and safe application protocols.

4. **Myth: DMSO Only Works as a Carrier for Other Substances**
   While DMSO is indeed an excellent carrier that can increase the effectiveness of other treatments, it is also a powerful therapeutic agent in its own right. Its analgesic, anti-inflammatory, and antioxidant properties make it highly beneficial even when used alone.

5. **Myth: DMSO Causes Irreversible Side Effects**
   DMSO has a relatively mild side-effect profile when used correctly. Side effects such as skin irritation or garlic-like odour

are usually temporary and manageable. Adverse effects are rare and generally occur when DMSO is used inappropriately or in very high concentrations.

The Science Behind DMSO

Understanding the science behind DMSO (Dimethyl Sulfoxide) is essential to appreciate its unique properties, mechanisms, and potential health benefits. In this section, we'll explore the chemistry and origins of DMSO, how it works in the body, the cellular mechanisms that enable it to reduce inflammation and pain, and the scientific research supporting its various applications. This science-based foundation aims to give you confidence in using DMSO as a natural treatment for a range of health conditions.

Chemistry and Origins of DMSO

DMSO, or Dimethyl Sulfoxide, is an organosulfur compound with the chemical formula $(CH_3)_2SO$. It was originally discovered as a byproduct of the wood pulp industry in the 19th century and subsequently developed into a versatile chemical compound with diverse applications. The structure of DMSO consists of two methyl groups (CH_3) attached to a central sulphur atom, which is further bonded to an oxygen atom. This molecular arrangement gives DMSO several unique properties:

1. **Solvent Properties**: DMSO is a polar aprotic solvent, meaning it can dissolve both polar and nonpolar substances. This property enables it to mix with a wide range of compounds, making it useful for dissolving various medications and herbal extracts for enhanced delivery into the body.
2. **Penetration and Carrier Ability**: DMSO can penetrate biological membranes such as skin and cell walls, a rare quality that allows it to act as a carrier for other

compounds, transporting them into tissues where they can be more effective. This characteristic has led to its use in delivering medications topically and transdermally, as DMSO enhances the absorption and effectiveness of many therapeutic substances.

3. **Chemical Stability**: DMSO is chemically stable under normal conditions, allowing it to be used in a wide range of temperatures and environmental conditions without breaking down or losing efficacy. This stability adds to its versatility and reliability in therapeutic applications.

DMSO's origin as a wood-derived compound aligns it with natural sources, which makes it appealing for alternative and holistic treatments. However, its chemical properties and synthesis methods have since evolved, allowing for purer and more refined forms suitable for medical and therapeutic use.

How DMSO Works in the Body

DMSO's ability to influence the body's healing processes is rooted in its unique physical and chemical properties. When applied topically or taken internally in controlled doses, DMSO interacts with cells and tissues in multiple ways, providing therapeutic effects that are both broad and profound. Here's an overview of how DMSO functions within the body:

1. **Rapid Absorption and Transport**: One of the most notable characteristics of DMSO is its ability to penetrate the skin and other biological membranes with ease. Unlike many substances that only affect surface tissues, DMSO can reach underlying tissues and even enter the bloodstream. This property allows it to act quickly, delivering relief and accelerating healing in targeted areas.

2. **Free Radical Scavenging**: DMSO is an antioxidant, meaning it helps neutralise free radicals—unstable molecules that can cause cellular damage and accelerate

ageing and disease. By binding to these free radicals, DMSO helps reduce oxidative stress and protects tissues from inflammation, degeneration, and other forms of damage caused by oxidative stress.

3. **Anti-Inflammatory Actions**: Inflammation is a major factor in many chronic conditions, from arthritis to muscle injuries. DMSO inhibits certain inflammatory processes at the cellular level, reducing the production of inflammatory cytokines and other signalling molecules that contribute to pain, swelling, and tissue damage.

4. **Improving Circulation**: DMSO promotes microcirculation by dilating blood vessels, which enhances oxygen and nutrient delivery to tissues. Improved blood flow also aids in the removal of cellular waste and toxins, further supporting tissue healing and recovery.

5. **Pain Relief and Nerve Modulation**: DMSO acts as an analgesic, providing

pain relief by modulating the transmission of pain signals along nerve pathways. This effect is particularly useful in treating conditions involving nerve pain, joint pain, and soft tissue injuries.

6. **Cell Membrane Stabilisation**: DMSO's action on cell membranes helps stabilise and protect cells, which can prevent cellular injury and improve cell survival in stressful or damaged tissues. By maintaining cellular integrity, DMSO supports overall tissue health and resilience.

Cellular Mechanisms: How DMSO Reduces Inflammation and Pain

DMSO's effects on inflammation and pain reduction are among its most powerful and well-documented benefits. These mechanisms operate at the cellular level, addressing the root causes of pain and inflammation rather than merely masking symptoms. Here's a closer look at how DMSO works on a cellular level to relieve inflammation and pain:

1. **Inhibition of Pro-Inflammatory Enzymes**: DMSO blocks the activity of certain enzymes and signalling molecules that drive the inflammatory response. For example, DMSO inhibits prostaglandins and leukotrienes—chemicals that cause inflammation and pain in response to injury or infection. By dampening these inflammatory mediators, DMSO reduces the redness, swelling, and pain commonly associated with inflammation.

2. **Reduction of Cytokine Release**: Cytokines are signalling molecules that play a crucial role in immune response and inflammation. In conditions like arthritis, elevated cytokine levels contribute to chronic inflammation and tissue damage. DMSO reduces the release of pro-inflammatory cytokines such as interleukins and tumour necrosis factor-alpha (TNF-α), thereby limiting

chronic inflammation and the resulting tissue destruction.

3. **Stabilisation of Cell Membranes**: When cells are damaged, they release inflammatory substances into surrounding tissues, exacerbating pain and swelling. DMSO stabilises cell membranes, preventing the release of these damaging substances. This stabilisation helps protect tissues from further damage and limits the inflammatory response in injured areas.

4. **Blocking Pain Transmission at the Nerve Level**: DMSO has an analgesic effect on nerve cells, which helps block the transmission of pain signals to the brain. This effect occurs due to DMSO's interaction with nerve fibres, which helps "numb" the area and provides relief from both acute and chronic pain. This nerve-modulating property is particularly beneficial for conditions involving nerve pain, such as neuropathy or sciatica.

5. **Enhanced Cellular Metabolism**: By improving cellular respiration and

enhancing ATP production, DMSO supports cellular metabolism, which is essential for tissue repair and regeneration. Cells with higher metabolic activity are better equipped to heal and recover from injury, reducing pain and accelerating recovery.

Through these mechanisms, DMSO works synergistically with the body's natural healing processes to reduce inflammation and pain effectively, without the need for synthetic drugs or invasive treatments.

Scientific Research and Clinical Studies

DMSO has been the subject of significant scientific research and clinical trials since the mid-20th century. Although it has faced some regulatory challenges, studies across the globe have demonstrated its effectiveness in various medical and therapeutic applications. Here are some key areas of research that validate DMSO's role in health and medicine:

1. **Pain Management and Arthritis**: Numerous studies have documented DMSO's effectiveness in reducing pain, particularly in patients with osteoarthritis and rheumatoid arthritis. A clinical trial published in *Arthritis & Rheumatism* showed that DMSO reduced pain and improved joint function in patients with arthritis, confirming its potential as a natural alternative to conventional pain medications.

2. **Anti-Inflammatory Effects**: Inflammation is a critical factor in many chronic diseases, and DMSO's anti-inflammatory properties have been widely studied. A study published in *Inflammation Research* found that DMSO reduced inflammatory markers in animal models, leading to decreased swelling and tissue damage. These findings support its

use in managing inflammatory conditions, including tendonitis and muscle injuries.

3. **Use in Bladder Conditions**: DMSO is FDA-approved for the treatment of interstitial cystitis, a chronic bladder condition characterised by pain and inflammation. Clinical studies, including those published in *Urology*, have demonstrated DMSO's ability to reduce bladder inflammation and alleviate the discomfort associated with interstitial cystitis.

4. **Skin and Tissue Healing**: Research in dermatology has shown that DMSO promotes wound healing, reduces scar formation, and alleviates burns. A study in *The Journal of Dermatology* documented the efficacy of DMSO in accelerating skin recovery and reducing the risk of infection in burn patients, further underscoring its value in skin care and wound management.

5. **Neurological Protection**: DMSO's neuroprotective properties have been

explored in several studies focused on spinal cord injury and traumatic brain injury. Research published in *Neurochemical Research* highlighted DMSO's role in reducing oxidative stress and preventing neuronal damage, which could make it useful for treating conditions involving nerve injury and neurological inflammation.

6. **Cardiovascular Benefits**: Preliminary studies indicate that DMSO may support cardiovascular health by improving blood flow, reducing blood viscosity, and acting as an antioxidant. Research in *Cardiovascular Research* suggests that DMSO's ability to enhance circulation and reduce oxidative stress may provide cardiovascular benefits, although more studies are needed to confirm these findings.

7. **Cancer Research**: While still in early stages, some research has examined DMSO's potential in cancer treatment, particularly as a drug carrier and

anti-inflammatory agent. Studies have shown that DMSO can enhance the effectiveness of certain chemotherapy drugs and reduce inflammation in cancer patients. However, this is an emerging area of research and warrants further investigation.

History and Discovery of DMSO

The story of Dimethyl Sulfoxide, commonly known as DMSO, is a fascinating journey that stretches from its accidental discovery as an industrial byproduct to its current recognition as a versatile therapeutic agent. The history of DMSO encompasses diverse stages, including its origins in industrial chemistry, its experimental journey in medical research, and its complex legal and regulatory trajectory worldwide.

The Origins and Early Uses

DMSO was first discovered in 1866 by Russian scientist Alexander Zaytsev, a chemist who was researching sulphur-containing compounds. At that time, DMSO was largely regarded as a chemical curiosity rather than a practical substance. It was derived from lignin, an organic compound found in wood pulp. As the paper and wood-processing industries grew, DMSO became more available as a byproduct, although its applications remained limited and largely industrial.

By the early 20th century, DMSO found its initial uses as an industrial solvent due to its remarkable ability to dissolve both polar and nonpolar substances. In industries such as pharmaceuticals, chemicals, and agriculture, it was prized for its non-toxic nature and versatility, especially for its capacity to dissolve compounds that other solvents could not. Despite its industrial value, however, DMSO was not recognized for its potential in health and medicine until much later.

In the 1950s, Dr. Stanley Jacob, a surgeon and medical researcher at Oregon Health & Science University, began studying DMSO's properties and potential therapeutic applications. Dr. Jacob observed that DMSO could penetrate the skin and transport other substances with it, a unique characteristic that sparked his interest in exploring its medical potential. His work with DMSO would eventually catalyse a new field of study in the treatment of pain, inflammation, and other ailments, leading to widespread use and both scientific and regulatory controversy.

Development in Medical Research

Dr. Stanley Jacob is often credited as the "Father of DMSO" due to his pioneering research in the medical applications of this compound. In the late 1950s and early 1960s, Dr. Jacob and his colleagues began investigating DMSO's potential as a medical treatment. Their work revealed several unexpected and promising effects of DMSO, including its ability to relieve pain, reduce inflammation, and promote healing when applied topically. These initial findings drew considerable attention, as DMSO offered a novel approach to managing various conditions without the side effects associated with conventional drugs.

Key Medical Discoveries and Applications

1. **Pain Relief and Anti-Inflammatory Effects**: Early studies found that DMSO was effective in alleviating pain, particularly in conditions like arthritis, muscle strain, and soft tissue injuries. Researchers observed that DMSO could penetrate the skin and deliver pain-relieving benefits directly to affected tissues. Its anti-inflammatory properties further enhanced its appeal for managing chronic inflammatory conditions, which led to extensive experimentation in pain management.

2. **Antioxidant Properties**: DMSO was found to possess antioxidant effects, helping to neutralise free radicals that

contribute to cellular damage. This discovery opened doors for using DMSO to treat conditions associated with oxidative stress, such as degenerative diseases and inflammatory disorders. Researchers hypothesised that its antioxidant effect could slow the progression of certain diseases and promote cellular health.

3. **Cryopreservation**: One of the most groundbreaking applications of DMSO in the medical field came in the 1960s when it was discovered that DMSO could protect cells during freezing. Researchers found that DMSO prevented ice crystal formation within cells, a breakthrough that allowed it to be used in the cryopreservation of human tissues, including bone marrow, stem cells, and organs. DMSO's role in cryopreservation remains one of its most important contributions to medical science, enabling the storage and transport of biological materials for research and transplantation.

4. **Transdermal Drug Delivery**: DMSO's ability to penetrate the skin and carry other substances along with it became the foundation for its use as a transdermal carrier. Medical researchers explored DMSO as a means of delivering medications directly through the skin, bypassing the digestive system and allowing for targeted treatment. This approach proved effective for various medications, including anti-inflammatory drugs, painkillers, and even certain cancer treatments.

5. **Bladder Conditions**: Another notable development was the use of DMSO in treating interstitial cystitis, a chronic inflammatory condition of the bladder. Clinical trials showed that DMSO could be instilled into the bladder to reduce pain and inflammation, providing relief for patients with this otherwise difficult-to-treat condition. In 1978, the FDA approved DMSO as a treatment for interstitial cystitis, making it one of the

few regulatory endorsements of DMSO in the United States.

These advancements in research underscored DMSO's potential as a therapeutic agent, leading to a surge in studies throughout the 1960s and 1970s. However, as DMSO gained popularity in medical circles, regulatory agencies became increasingly concerned about its safety, especially due to the absence of large-scale clinical trials at that time.

Legal and Regulatory Status Worldwide

The regulatory history of DMSO is complex and often contradictory. Despite its promising effects in medical research, DMSO faced substantial obstacles in gaining widespread approval as a therapeutic agent. Much of the controversy surrounding DMSO stems from concerns about its safety and the limited understanding of its long-term effects on human health.

United States

In the U.S., DMSO's regulatory journey has been fraught with challenges. In the 1960s, the FDA temporarily halted all clinical trials involving DMSO due to concerns about potential side effects, specifically regarding changes in vision observed in some animal studies. Although subsequent studies in humans found no evidence of these side effects, the initial concerns cast a shadow over DMSO's reputation and slowed its acceptance as a medical treatment.

By 1978, however, the FDA approved DMSO for the treatment of interstitial cystitis. This approval remains one of the few FDA-endorsed uses of DMSO, and it has helped to cement DMSO's status in pain management and inflammation reduction in specific cases. Despite this limited approval, the FDA has been reluctant to endorse DMSO for broader medical uses, and its use in the U.S. has largely been limited to alternative medicine circles.

Europe and Canada

In Europe and Canada, DMSO has been more readily accepted, particularly in countries like Germany and Russia, where it is widely used for pain relief, inflammation, and other applications. In Germany, DMSO is commonly prescribed for musculoskeletal pain and joint disorders, while in Russia, it is considered a staple in the treatment of injuries, arthritis, and soft tissue pain. Health Canada has also allowed DMSO's use for specific medical conditions, and Canadian physicians sometimes prescribe it off-label for conditions like interstitial cystitis and chronic pain.

Other Parts of the World

In Asia and South America, DMSO has seen broader acceptance in both clinical and alternative medicine practices. In Japan, for instance, DMSO is used in both mainstream and integrative medicine for a variety of conditions, particularly for inflammation and pain management. In South America, DMSO has found a niche in alternative medicine practices, where it is commonly used for joint pain, muscle soreness, and wound healing.

Despite DMSO's approval and use in various countries, its legal status remains somewhat ambiguous and varies widely depending on local regulations. In some countries, it is available over the counter for topical use, while in others, it is restricted to prescription-only or banned outright due to safety concerns.

Current Regulatory Landscape and Future Prospects

Today, DMSO remains a regulated substance in many countries, with its use often restricted to specific medical applications or alternative therapies. However, ongoing research and increased public awareness have contributed to a resurgence of interest in DMSO, and there are calls within the scientific and medical communities for further studies to better understand its full range of therapeutic effects.

In recent years, as more evidence of DMSO's benefits has emerged, some regulatory agencies are re-evaluating their stance on the compound. Advocates for DMSO argue that with proper guidance on dosage and usage, it can be safely used for a broader range of conditions. Meanwhile, the compound's role in cryopreservation and its potential as a drug delivery system are increasingly recognized, opening new avenues for regulatory approval.

Properties and Benefits of DMSO

DMSO, or Dimethyl Sulfoxide, has a diverse range of properties that make it a unique and powerful therapeutic agent in both conventional and alternative medicine. As a natural compound derived from lignin in wood, DMSO is known for its impressive bioavailability, ability to penetrate biological membranes, and versatility in treating various ailments. Its properties span from powerful anti-inflammatory and analgesic effects to antioxidant and immune-boosting benefits. Additionally, DMSO's capability to support cellular health and facilitate healing has made it a focal point in treating chronic pain, inflammation, and even degenerative diseases.

Anti-Inflammatory and Analgesic Properties

One of the most celebrated attributes of DMSO is its powerful anti-inflammatory and analgesic (pain-relieving) properties. These effects make it especially valuable in managing conditions such as arthritis, muscle injuries, and chronic pain disorders. Unlike traditional anti-inflammatory drugs, which can have adverse effects on the stomach and liver, DMSO works topically and is generally well tolerated by most users.

How DMSO Reduces Inflammation

Inflammation is the body's natural response to injury or infection, but chronic inflammation can lead to persistent pain and tissue damage. DMSO mitigates inflammation by inhibiting the formation of inflammatory mediators, including prostaglandins and cytokines, which are chemicals that promote inflammation in the body. By reducing these mediators, DMSO helps to control the inflammatory response, alleviating pain and allowing the body to focus on healing rather than fighting prolonged inflammation.

DMSO also affects the migration of white blood cells to sites of inflammation. During inflammation, white blood cells congregate in affected areas, releasing enzymes that can exacerbate tissue damage. DMSO has been shown to limit this accumulation, thereby reducing tissue injury and promoting faster recovery. This makes it especially useful for conditions where inflammation is a significant contributor to pain and tissue damage, such as in arthritis and sports injuries.

DMSO as a Pain Reliever

DMSO's analgesic properties are another key benefit. Pain relief with DMSO is achieved through multiple mechanisms. First, DMSO interferes with nerve conduction by stabilising cell membranes, which helps reduce pain signals sent to the brain. This action is particularly effective for localised pain, where DMSO can be applied directly to the skin over the painful area for rapid relief.

Additionally, DMSO's ability to penetrate tissues allows it to reach deeper layers, such as muscles and joints, where it can address underlying causes of pain more effectively than many topical treatments. This makes it an excellent option for people suffering from musculoskeletal pain, including back pain, muscle spasms, and joint pain associated with conditions like osteoarthritis and rheumatoid arthritis.

Clinical Uses of DMSO for Pain and Inflammation

Due to its efficacy in managing pain and inflammation, DMSO has been widely used in clinical settings for conditions like:

- **Arthritis**: Both osteoarthritis and rheumatoid arthritis benefit from DMSO's pain-relieving and anti-inflammatory effects. Applied topically, it can reduce joint pain and stiffness, providing relief to individuals struggling with these chronic conditions.

- **Soft Tissue Injuries**: DMSO is commonly used to treat strains, sprains, and bruises. Its penetration into soft tissues and muscles allows it to alleviate pain and speed up the healing process, making it a popular choice among athletes and individuals with physical injuries.
- **Headaches**: DMSO can also be applied to relieve tension headaches and migraines. Although the exact mechanism is not fully understood, it is believed to work by reducing inflammation in surrounding tissues and muscles.

Antioxidant and Immune-Boosting Benefits

DMSO has significant antioxidant properties, making it an excellent ally against oxidative stress, which is implicated in ageing, chronic diseases, and immune system suppression. Oxidative stress occurs when there is an imbalance between free radicals (unstable molecules) and antioxidants, leading to cellular damage. DMSO's antioxidant benefits are an important reason it's considered beneficial in the treatment and prevention of degenerative conditions and immune-related disorders.

How DMSO Works as an Antioxidant

As an antioxidant, DMSO has a unique ability to neutralise free radicals, the molecules responsible for causing cellular damage and accelerating the ageing process. Free radicals are produced in response to environmental stressors, infections, inflammation, and metabolic processes. When these unstable molecules interact with healthy cells, they can lead to damage at the cellular level, potentially contributing to diseases like heart disease, diabetes, cancer, and neurodegenerative disorders.

DMSO stabilises free radicals by donating electrons to these molecules, effectively neutralising them and preventing further cellular damage. By reducing the oxidative burden on the body, DMSO contributes to healthier cells and supports the body's natural repair mechanisms. This property is particularly beneficial in managing chronic inflammation, as oxidative stress and inflammation often go hand in hand, creating a cycle of damage and degradation in tissues and organs.

Immune-Boosting Properties of DMSO

DMSO also exhibits immune-boosting properties, which have been studied for their potential to support the body's natural defence systems. By reducing oxidative stress and inflammation, DMSO helps create an environment where the immune system can function optimally. Furthermore, some studies suggest that DMSO might enhance the activity of macrophages—immune cells that play a critical role in identifying and destroying pathogens in the body.

The immune-boosting benefits of DMSO may make it a valuable addition to protocols for individuals with compromised immune systems, such as those with chronic infections or autoimmune conditions. By supporting a balanced immune response, DMSO may help the body resist infections more effectively and promote overall immune resilience.

How DMSO Enhances Cellular Health

At a cellular level, DMSO has several unique effects that contribute to its therapeutic potential. Its structure allows it to penetrate cell membranes easily, which enables it to reach tissues that many other substances cannot. This cellular penetration facilitates a variety of health benefits, including improved nutrient absorption, better waste removal, and enhanced cellular repair mechanisms.

Cellular Penetration and Tissue Absorption

DMSO's small molecular size and polar structure make it exceptionally effective at penetrating cell membranes and diffusing into tissues. This property is one of the reasons DMSO is used as a carrier in drug delivery systems—it can bring other therapeutic agents along with it into cells, enhancing their absorption and efficacy. DMSO's penetration also means it can reach deeper layers of tissue, such as muscles, joints, and internal organs, delivering its benefits where they're most needed.

DMSO and Cellular Detoxification

One of the less well-known properties of DMSO is its ability to aid in cellular detoxification. By increasing cell membrane permeability, DMSO facilitates the removal of waste products and toxins from cells. This effect can be especially beneficial in conditions where toxin buildup contributes to pain and inflammation, such as chronic pain syndromes and fibromyalgia. DMSO's detoxifying effect may also enhance recovery from exercise, injury, and illness, supporting overall cellular health and vitality.

DMSO's Role in Cellular Repair and Regeneration

Studies have shown that DMSO promotes cellular repair and regeneration. It does this by stimulating fibroblasts, the cells responsible for producing collagen and other connective tissue components. Collagen is essential for tissue repair, providing structural integrity to the skin, muscles, and joints. By enhancing collagen production, DMSO helps support the body's natural healing processes, making it especially useful for wound healing, scar reduction, and tissue regeneration.

Additionally, DMSO has been shown to help stabilise the membranes of damaged cells, preventing further leakage of cellular contents and reducing additional tissue damage. This stabilising effect is beneficial in cases of trauma, injury, and inflammation, where cellular integrity is compromised.

DMSO as a Cellular Protector in Degenerative Diseases

Given its cellular health benefits, DMSO has been studied for its potential in managing degenerative diseases like Alzheimer's, Parkinson's, and multiple sclerosis. By reducing oxidative stress and inflammation, DMSO may help slow the progression of these conditions, although further research is needed to fully understand its effects in these cases. Its ability to reach the brain by crossing the blood-brain barrier further supports its potential for neurological health, as it may be able to alleviate some of the underlying cellular damage and inflammation associated with neurodegenerative diseases.

Forms and Concentrations of DMSO

DMSO is available in various forms and concentrations, each suited to different therapeutic needs and applications. Knowing which form and concentration to choose is essential for maximising the therapeutic potential of DMSO while minimising side effects and ensuring safe, effective use. This section looks into the most common forms—gel, liquid, and cream—along with guidelines on concentration and purity levels. Whether you're considering DMSO for topical use, mixing it with other compounds, or incorporating it into a healthcare regimen, this guide will help you select the best option for your needs.

Gel, Liquid, and Cream Forms

DMSO's versatility is reflected in the range of forms it comes in, including gels, liquids, and creams. Each form has distinct advantages depending on the intended application and area of the body it is applied to. Here's an in-depth look at each form:

1. Gel Form

DMSO in gel form is one of the most popular options, especially for those new to using DMSO for topical application. Gels are convenient to apply, easy to control, and have a thicker consistency than liquids, which makes them ideal for targeted areas such as joints, muscles, and specific areas of pain or inflammation. The gel form is less likely to drip or spread uncontrollably, allowing users to apply it precisely where they need it.

DMSO gel is often used for conditions that benefit from localised treatment, such as arthritis, muscle sprains, or bruises. It is usually applied in a thin layer directly to the skin, where it penetrates to relieve pain and inflammation in underlying tissues. Gels are also beneficial for treating skin conditions like acne, rosacea, and psoriasis, as they provide a controlled release that can reduce irritation while maximising the benefits of DMSO.

Additionally, many DMSO gels are formulated with other beneficial ingredients, such as aloe vera or certain essential oils, which enhance their soothing and healing properties. However, for those with sensitive skin, it's essential to check for added ingredients, as some may cause irritation.

2. Liquid Form

The liquid form of DMSO is the most concentrated and versatile option available. Liquid DMSO has a high bioavailability, meaning it's rapidly absorbed into the skin and tissues. Because it's in liquid form, it can be easily diluted to reach the desired concentration for various uses. Liquid DMSO is particularly effective when a more extensive application is needed or when users need to adjust the concentration based on sensitivity or therapeutic needs.

Liquid DMSO is commonly used for mixing with other substances, such as essential oils, saline solutions, or even prescription medications, where it acts as a carrier to facilitate the penetration of these substances into the tissues. Due to its rapid penetration, it is also used in higher-concentration applications, where stronger effects are needed—such as in sports medicine or for treating chronic, severe pain.

The downside of liquid DMSO is that it can be difficult to control and may spread more than gels or creams, potentially affecting unintended areas. This is especially important to consider when using higher concentrations, as accidental application to unintended skin areas or eyes can cause irritation or mild burning. Many users find it helpful to use a small dropper or spray bottle to control the application more precisely.

3. Cream Form

DMSO in cream form is similar to gel but has a lighter texture and is generally less concentrated, making it a more gentle option. Creams are often preferred for sensitive skin and delicate areas, such as the face or thin skin regions. The creamy consistency allows for a slower release of DMSO, reducing the likelihood of any stinging or burning sensation that might occur with the more concentrated gel or liquid forms.

Creams are often formulated with moisturising agents like lanolin, aloe vera, or coconut oil to counteract any drying effect of DMSO. This makes them an excellent choice for individuals with dry or sensitive skin, as well as for those seeking a milder application experience. The cream form is also preferred for cosmetic applications, such as minimising scars or reducing skin inflammation, where a gentle and hydrating product is beneficial.

Due to its mildness, DMSO cream is frequently used for skin rejuvenation purposes, and it may be applied as part of a daily skincare routine. The cream's soothing properties also make it popular among individuals looking to use DMSO for minor skin conditions, such as eczema or irritation, without experiencing the intensity of a liquid or gel.

Concentration Guidelines and Purity Levels

Choosing the right concentration of DMSO is essential for both safety and efficacy. DMSO concentrations typically range from as low as 10% to 99%, depending on the intended use, skin sensitivity, and the area of application. Here's a closer look at concentration options and guidelines on purity levels:

Typical Concentration Ranges

1. **Low Concentrations (10-30%)**: Low concentrations are generally recommended for people with sensitive

skin, younger individuals, or when using DMSO for delicate areas of the body, such as the face or neck. At these levels, DMSO can still deliver beneficial effects without overwhelming the skin or causing significant irritation. Low concentrations are also ideal for mild conditions such as minor cuts, scrapes, or inflammation.

2. **Moderate Concentrations (40-70%)**: This range is one of the most common concentrations used for general applications, such as treating joint pain, muscle aches, and localised inflammation. Moderate concentrations strike a balance between efficacy and tolerance, offering enough potency to address pain and inflammation without causing too much irritation. They are commonly used in gels and creams that are applied to larger areas, such as the back, shoulders, or knees.

3. **High Concentrations (80-99%)**: High concentrations are typically reserved for cases requiring intense pain relief or deep penetration, such as in severe arthritis or

chronic musculoskeletal issues. These concentrations should be used cautiously, as they are more likely to cause skin reactions or a burning sensation, especially for individuals with sensitive skin. High-concentration DMSO is often diluted for use or mixed with other carrier agents to improve tolerability.

Purity Levels

Purity is crucial when choosing DMSO, as impure products can introduce contaminants that may cause irritation or even negate the therapeutic benefits. DMSO purity is generally rated in three levels:

1. **Pharmaceutical Grade (99.9% Pure)**: This is the highest level of purity available and is recommended for therapeutic applications, especially when DMSO is intended for medicinal use on sensitive areas of the body. Pharmaceutical-grade DMSO has been refined to remove impurities and contaminants, making it

safer for human application. This grade is generally preferred for direct skin application or when mixing DMSO with other therapeutic agents.

2. **Industrial Grade**: Industrial-grade DMSO has a lower purity level and may contain impurities that make it unsuitable for therapeutic use. This grade is typically used in industrial applications, such as manufacturing, and is not recommended for personal use or medical purposes. Industrial-grade DMSO may contain residues or contaminants from the manufacturing process that can cause skin irritation or other adverse effects.

3. **Lab Grade**: Lab-grade DMSO falls between pharmaceutical and industrial grades in terms of purity. While it may be cleaner than industrial-grade DMSO, it is still not as pure as pharmaceutical-grade. Lab-grade DMSO can sometimes be used for topical applications, but it is not guaranteed to be free of impurities that could irritate the skin.

How to Choose the Right Form and Concentration for Your Needs

Choosing the right DMSO form and concentration depends on your intended use, skin sensitivity, and desired therapeutic effects. Here are a few guidelines to help you make an informed decision:

1. **For General Pain and Inflammation**: If you're looking to treat muscle pain, joint inflammation, or arthritis, a gel or cream form with a moderate concentration (50-70%) is usually effective. These forms are easy to apply, and the moderate concentration provides potent pain relief without excessive irritation.

2. **For Sensitive Skin or Cosmetic Applications**: Individuals with sensitive skin or those applying DMSO to the face should opt for cream-based DMSO with a lower concentration (10-30%). Creams are gentler on the skin, while low

concentrations reduce the risk of irritation. This form is also suitable for cosmetic purposes, such as scar reduction or skin rejuvenation.

3. **For Severe Pain or Deep Tissue Penetration**: In cases where deep penetration is required, such as with severe arthritis or sports injuries, high-concentration liquid DMSO (80-99%) can be effective. However, these concentrations should be used with caution, preferably diluted with water or a carrier oil, to minimise the risk of skin irritation.

4. **When Mixing DMSO with Other Agents**: Liquid DMSO is preferred for mixing with other therapeutic agents, as it can serve as an effective carrier. Concentrations in the 50-70% range are typically adequate for facilitating penetration of other compounds while minimising potential irritation from the DMSO itself.

5. **For Immune or Systemic Benefits**: If you are considering DMSO for systemic benefits, such as boosting immune function or providing antioxidant support, lower concentrations applied consistently over larger areas may be beneficial. Consult with a healthcare provider to determine the best approach for your specific health goals.

DMSO for Pain Management

DMSO (Dimethyl Sulfoxide) has gained popularity as a versatile and effective option for managing various types of pain. With its unique properties that allow it to penetrate tissues deeply, reduce inflammation, and enhance blood circulation, DMSO has become a natural alternative for those seeking relief from conditions such as joint pain, muscle pain, arthritis, migraines, chronic headaches, and even post-surgical recovery.

Treating Joint Pain, Muscle Pain, and Arthritis

One of the most prominent uses of DMSO is for alleviating joint and muscle pain, especially in conditions such as arthritis. DMSO's anti-inflammatory and analgesic properties make it particularly effective for reducing the swelling, stiffness, and discomfort associated with joint and muscle pain. Here's a closer look at how DMSO can be utilised for these conditions:

Joint Pain Relief

Joint pain can result from various causes, including injury, overuse, and chronic conditions like osteoarthritis and rheumatoid arthritis. DMSO is especially effective for joint pain because it penetrates deep into the tissues, targeting the source of inflammation and discomfort. When applied topically to the affected joint, DMSO works to inhibit the release of pro-inflammatory cytokines—molecules that signal inflammation in the body—thereby reducing pain and swelling.

DMSO also promotes improved blood flow to the area, which enhances the delivery of oxygen and nutrients to the joint. This circulation boost can expedite healing, relieve stiffness, and provide long-lasting relief, making it an excellent choice for individuals struggling with joint-related discomfort.

Muscle Pain Relief

Muscle pain, often caused by strain, injury, or conditions like fibromyalgia, can significantly affect mobility and quality of life. DMSO's pain-relieving properties work well on sore muscles because it relaxes muscle tissue, improves blood flow, and reduces lactic acid buildup. By breaking down lactic acid—the chemical responsible for post-exercise soreness—DMSO can speed up recovery after intense physical activity or injury.

Athletes often turn to DMSO gels or creams after training to reduce muscle inflammation, relieve pain, and promote quicker recovery. Because it's a natural product, DMSO is also a popular choice for individuals who prefer to avoid pharmaceutical painkillers, which can carry unwanted side effects.

Arthritis Management

Arthritis, especially osteoarthritis and rheumatoid arthritis, is one of the most common applications for DMSO in pain management. People with arthritis experience chronic inflammation of the joints, leading to pain, reduced flexibility, and even deformity over time. DMSO offers a dual-action benefit for arthritis sufferers: it reduces inflammation in the joint and relieves pain at the site. When applied to affected areas, DMSO can bring relief within minutes, with effects that last several hours.

In some cases, patients with rheumatoid arthritis (an autoimmune condition) have reported reduced swelling and improved joint function with regular DMSO applications. It's essential, however, to use the appropriate concentration of DMSO for arthritis treatment to avoid skin irritation, particularly for those with sensitive skin. Many users find that a concentration between 50% and 70% provides sufficient relief without causing irritation.

Relief for Migraines and Chronic Headaches

Migraines and chronic headaches are debilitating conditions that impact millions of people worldwide. Conventional treatments often involve medication, which may come with side effects or lack effectiveness over time. DMSO, however, provides a unique alternative for migraine sufferers by addressing the inflammation and vascular factors that contribute to these painful episodes.

How DMSO Works for Migraines

Migraines are believed to result from a combination of neurological and vascular changes, often including dilation of blood vessels in the brain and an inflammatory response. DMSO has the unique ability to penetrate the blood-brain barrier, which allows it to directly affect the inflammation and blood flow in the brain.

When applied topically around the neck, temples, or forehead, DMSO can relieve pressure caused by vascular dilation and reduce the inflammatory response associated with migraines. By relaxing the blood vessels and improving circulation, DMSO can alleviate the intensity and duration of migraine attacks. Additionally, its analgesic effect provides immediate relief from pain, which is especially beneficial during the acute phase of a migraine.

Reducing the Frequency of Chronic Headaches

For individuals suffering from chronic headaches, regular DMSO use may reduce both the frequency and severity of episodes. Headaches often stem from tension, muscular strain, or inflammation, all of which DMSO can address effectively. Applying DMSO to areas of muscular tension, such as the shoulders and neck, can release tight muscles, improve blood flow, and reduce the trigger points that may lead to headaches.

Many users incorporate DMSO into their routine at the first sign of a headache, as it can help stop the progression of symptoms before they develop into a full-blown migraine or severe headache. However, it is important to avoid applying DMSO directly near the eyes, as the vapours may cause irritation.

Post-Surgical and Injury Recovery

DMSO has long been used in sports medicine and physical therapy for post-surgical and injury recovery. Whether from surgery, accidents, or athletic injuries, the pain and inflammation associated with tissue damage can be effectively managed with DMSO.

Role of DMSO in Healing and Recovery

DMSO's primary mechanism of action in post-surgical recovery lies in its ability to reduce inflammation and enhance blood circulation. Following surgery or injury, inflammation is a natural response, but excessive inflammation can delay healing and increase pain. By inhibiting inflammatory pathways, DMSO reduces swelling and promotes a faster, more comfortable recovery.

Additionally, DMSO's role as a carrier substance means it can be combined with other therapeutic agents, such as certain pain-relieving or anti-inflammatory medications. When used as a carrier, DMSO allows these medications to penetrate tissues more effectively, providing targeted relief without needing high doses.

Muscle and Tendon Injury

For muscle strains, sprains, tendon injuries, and ligament tears, DMSO can play a significant role in reducing recovery time and managing pain. It is particularly popular among athletes for its ability to alleviate pain from common sports injuries, such as tennis elbow, plantar fasciitis, and rotator cuff tears. When applied to an injured area, DMSO quickly penetrates the skin, reaching deeper tissue layers, reducing pain and speeding up the body's natural repair mechanisms.

In cases of severe injury, DMSO may be used in combination with physical therapy for optimal recovery. The anti-inflammatory effects of DMSO not only aid in pain relief but also improve mobility, making physical therapy less painful and more effective.

Post-Surgical Scarring and Tissue Repair

DMSO also has applications in reducing scarring, a common concern for individuals recovering from surgery. It aids in scar tissue breakdown and promotes healthy skin regrowth, which can be beneficial for both cosmetic reasons and functional recovery. Scar tissue can sometimes impair mobility or lead to chronic pain, and regular DMSO application can help soften and diminish these adhesions over time.

For surgical incisions, DMSO should be applied once the wound has fully closed to avoid any risk of infection. Users often start with a lower concentration to test skin tolerance before moving to a moderate or high concentration for scar management.

Safety Tips for Using DMSO for Pain Management

1. **Patch Testing**: Before applying DMSO widely, it's wise to do a patch test on a small area of skin to check for any sensitivity or allergic reaction.
2. **Gradual Increase**: Start with lower concentrations if you're new to DMSO and gradually increase as your skin and body acclimate.
3. **Avoid Open Wounds**: DMSO should not be applied to open wounds or broken skin, as it may increase the risk of infection.
4. **Consultation with a Professional**: Individuals with chronic conditions, or

those who are recovering from surgery, should consult their healthcare provider before using DMSO, especially if they are on other medications.

5. **Avoid the Eye Area**: When using DMSO on the face or for headaches, avoid the eyes, as the vapours can be irritating.

DMSO for Skin and Wound Healing

Dimethyl Sulfoxide (DMSO) is widely recognized for its benefits in pain relief and anti-inflammatory effects, but its applications in skin and wound healing are equally significant. DMSO's unique ability to penetrate the skin barrier and promote cellular repair makes it an exceptional aid for treating cuts, scrapes, burns, bruising, swelling, scars, and various skin conditions. By targeting inflammation, enhancing blood flow, and supporting collagen production, DMSO accelerates the body's natural healing processes, making it an excellent addition to any wound care regimen.

Treating Cuts, Scrapes, and Burns

Injuries to the skin, such as cuts, scrapes, and burns, are among the most common types of wounds that can benefit from DMSO treatment. The skin serves as the body's first line of defence against infection, so healing these injuries quickly and effectively is crucial to maintaining overall health. DMSO's properties not only reduce pain and inflammation but also aid in faster tissue repair, making it a useful addition to first-aid treatments.

How DMSO Aids Wound Healing

DMSO's capacity to deeply penetrate tissues allows it to reach damaged cells quickly, delivering its therapeutic effects to the injury site almost immediately. When applied to cuts or scrapes, DMSO works by reducing inflammation in the affected area, thereby minimising redness, pain, and swelling. It also promotes better blood circulation, which enhances the supply of nutrients and oxygen to the wound, accelerating the healing process.

In the case of burns, DMSO helps soothe the pain and reduce the risk of blistering. DMSO's cooling effect can bring immediate relief to the burning sensation and mitigate tissue damage if applied shortly after the injury. Additionally, DMSO has been shown to prevent cell death in thermal burns by stabilising cellular membranes and reducing oxidative stress. Applying a gel or diluted liquid form of DMSO to burns can lessen the severity of the injury, reduce scarring, and promote faster healing.

Recommended Application for Minor Wounds

For treating minor cuts, scrapes, or burns with DMSO, it is important to use a form that's gentle on the skin, such as a gel or a low-concentration liquid. Here's a general guide on how to apply DMSO for minor skin injuries:

1. **Clean the Wound First**: Always clean the wound thoroughly with water and mild soap to remove any debris or bacteria before applying DMSO.
2. **Dilute if Necessary**: Use a diluted DMSO solution (typically around 50% or lower concentration) for sensitive skin, especially for burns or open wounds. Applying undiluted DMSO to an open wound may cause irritation.
3. **Apply Gently**: Apply a thin layer of DMSO gel or liquid to the wound area using clean hands or a sterile applicator. Avoid excessive rubbing, as this could aggravate the injury.
4. **Cover if Needed**: In some cases, covering the wound with a sterile bandage after applying DMSO can help protect the area from further irritation and contamination.
5. **Frequency**: Apply DMSO 1-2 times daily until the wound shows significant improvement, typically within a few days.

DMSO in Managing Scars and Skin Conditions

One of DMSO's lesser-known applications is in the management of scars and various skin conditions. Due to its ability to support collagen production, reduce inflammation, and improve blood flow, DMSO can be an effective solution for reducing scar tissue, improving skin texture, and even managing certain skin ailments like eczema and psoriasis.

Reducing Scarring and Enhancing Skin Regeneration

Scarring is a natural part of the healing process, but in some cases, scars can become raised, thickened, or discoloured, leading to aesthetic and functional concerns. DMSO promotes the breakdown of collagen fibres that cause excessive scarring, softening and flattening scar tissue over time. It also helps regenerate new, healthy skin cells by increasing blood circulation to the affected area, which delivers nutrients necessary for skin repair.

Regular application of DMSO to scars can also improve the flexibility of the surrounding skin, making it particularly beneficial for scars that limit movement or feel tight. Users often report noticeable improvements in the appearance of both fresh and older scars after several weeks of consistent DMSO use. For best results, DMSO should be applied to scar tissue regularly—often 1-2 times a day—while avoiding irritation by using a low to moderate concentration (50-70%).

Treating Skin Conditions: Eczema, Psoriasis, and Acne

DMSO has shown promise in alleviating symptoms of chronic skin conditions like eczema, psoriasis, and acne. These conditions are often driven by underlying inflammation, immune response, or bacterial factors, and DMSO's anti-inflammatory, antimicrobial, and immune-modulating properties make it highly suitable for addressing these root causes.

- **Eczema and Psoriasis**: These skin conditions involve inflammation and often manifest as red, itchy, and flaky patches. Applying DMSO to affected areas can soothe inflammation, reduce itchiness, and help restore moisture balance in the skin. DMSO may also reduce the autoimmune response associated with these conditions, making it effective in minimising flare-ups.

- **Acne**: DMSO's antimicrobial properties allow it to address acne-causing bacteria on the skin, while its anti-inflammatory effects help reduce redness and swelling. Since it enhances skin penetration, DMSO can be used in combination with other topical acne treatments to improve their effectiveness, though care should be taken to avoid irritation.

Reducing Bruising and Swelling

Bruising and swelling can result from injury, surgical procedures, or conditions like venous insufficiency. When applied topically, DMSO reduces bruising and swelling by targeting inflammation, improving circulation, and aiding in the body's natural repair mechanisms. The result is faster recovery from trauma, with less visible bruising and reduced discomfort.

Mechanism of Action: How DMSO Reduces Bruising

Bruises occur when small blood vessels under the skin break and blood pools in surrounding tissue. This results in the familiar discoloration, tenderness, and swelling associated with bruising. DMSO's ability to increase blood flow and promote the reabsorption of trapped blood particles accelerates the fading of bruises. Furthermore, its anti-inflammatory properties work to prevent excessive swelling and reduce tenderness.

Applying DMSO to bruised areas not only helps disperse the pooled blood but also stimulates local circulation, allowing the body to process and heal the affected tissue more quickly. Individuals who use DMSO for bruising often report that bruises fade within days instead of weeks, and the pain associated with bruises subsides almost immediately.

Effective Application for Bruising and Swelling

To use DMSO for treating bruises and swelling, follow these steps:

1. **Clean the Skin**: Before application, ensure the skin is clean to avoid introducing any contaminants that could increase irritation.
2. **Use a Lower Concentration**: For sensitive or tender areas, especially on the face or where the skin is thin, start with a 50% DMSO concentration to prevent irritation.
3. **Apply a Thin Layer**: Gently rub a small amount of DMSO gel or liquid on the bruised area without excessive pressure. Allow the DMSO to be absorbed naturally.

4. **Frequency**: Apply DMSO once or twice daily, especially in the initial days following the injury, to reduce swelling and speed up the healing process.

5. **Avoid Broken Skin**: Do not apply DMSO to areas where the skin is broken, as it can cause irritation if it enters an open wound.

Considerations for Safe and Effective Use of DMSO in Skin and Wound Healing

When using DMSO for skin and wound healing, it's important to keep a few key considerations in mind to ensure safety and effectiveness:

- **Concentration Levels**: The concentration of DMSO should be appropriate for the specific application and skin sensitivity. Lower concentrations (50% or below) are suitable for delicate areas or open wounds, while higher concentrations may be used on less sensitive areas or for scar management.

- **Patch Testing**: As with any topical application, patch testing DMSO on a small area of skin can help determine if you are sensitive to it. Some people may experience minor irritation, so testing first can prevent discomfort.

- **Avoid Use Near Eyes**: DMSO should not be applied near the eyes or mucous membranes, as it can cause stinging and discomfort.

- **Hygiene**: Ensure your hands and the application area are clean before applying DMSO to prevent introducing any contaminants, as DMSO readily absorbs and can carry substances through the skin barrier.

DMSO for Inflammation and Autoimmune Disorders

Inflammation and autoimmune disorders are some of the most common health challenges people face today. From chronic pain and joint stiffness to systemic immune responses, these conditions often require long-term management strategies. Dimethyl Sulfoxide (DMSO) has emerged as a natural, effective alternative for managing inflammation and certain autoimmune disorders. This versatile substance is gaining recognition for its ability to reduce swelling, alleviate pain, and enhance healing processes, providing relief for a range of inflammatory and autoimmune conditions. In this section, we will explain how DMSO can be used to manage rheumatoid arthritis, osteoarthritis, tendonitis, bursitis, fibromyalgia, lupus, and other similar conditions.

Managing Rheumatoid Arthritis and Osteoarthritis

Rheumatoid arthritis (RA) and osteoarthritis (OA) are among the most common inflammatory joint diseases, affecting millions worldwide. Both conditions are marked by pain, stiffness, and limited mobility, making daily activities difficult for sufferers. DMSO has been studied for its potential to alleviate symptoms of these conditions, offering a natural solution for pain and inflammation relief.

Rheumatoid Arthritis (RA)

Rheumatoid arthritis is an autoimmune disease where the body's immune system mistakenly attacks healthy joint tissue, leading to inflammation, pain, and potential joint damage. DMSO's anti-inflammatory and analgesic properties make it a useful treatment option for individuals suffering from RA. When applied topically, DMSO penetrates the skin and tissues, reducing inflammation in the affected joints and providing pain relief. It also has the ability to increase blood circulation, which helps deliver oxygen and nutrients to damaged tissues, speeding up the healing process.

How DMSO Helps in RA:

1. **Pain Relief**: DMSO is a powerful analgesic that helps reduce joint pain associated with RA. By modulating pain perception, it can provide significant relief, especially when used in combination with other treatments.
2. **Reducing Swelling**: DMSO's anti-inflammatory effects help decrease the swelling in affected joints, improving

mobility and reducing stiffness. This can be particularly beneficial during flare-ups of RA when inflammation is at its peak.

3. **Inhibiting Inflammatory Enzymes**: DMSO has been shown to inhibit the production of certain enzymes and proteins that promote inflammation, such as cyclooxygenase (COX), which plays a role in joint inflammation.

Osteoarthritis (OA)

Osteoarthritis, on the other hand, is a degenerative joint disease characterised by the breakdown of cartilage and the resulting pain and inflammation in the joints. While OA does not involve an autoimmune response like RA, it still involves significant inflammation that can be debilitating. DMSO's ability to penetrate deep into tissues and reduce both pain and inflammation makes it an ideal option for managing OA symptoms.

How DMSO Helps in OA:

1. **Joint Lubrication**: DMSO has been found to help improve joint lubrication, which can reduce friction and ease movement in affected joints, such as the knees, hips, and spine.

2. **Anti-Inflammatory Action**: By reducing the levels of inflammatory markers in the body, DMSO helps to alleviate the swelling and discomfort that comes with OA, especially in the early stages of the disease.

3. **Cartilage Protection**: Research suggests that DMSO may help protect cartilage from further damage by promoting tissue regeneration and reducing oxidative stress.

Relief for Tendonitis and Bursitis

Tendonitis and bursitis are conditions that cause inflammation in the tendons and bursae, respectively, often leading to pain, swelling, and reduced range of motion. These conditions are typically caused by overuse, repetitive motion, or trauma to the affected area. DMSO has been shown to be effective in reducing the pain and inflammation associated with both tendonitis and bursitis, speeding up the healing process and restoring mobility.

Tendonitis

Tendonitis is the inflammation of a tendon, usually resulting from repetitive strain or overuse. Common sites for tendonitis include the shoulder, elbow, knee, and wrist. DMSO can help to ease the pain and swelling associated with tendonitis by targeting the root cause—inflammation.

How DMSO Helps with Tendonitis:

1. **Pain Reduction**: DMSO's analgesic properties work quickly to reduce pain, making it easier to engage in daily activities without discomfort.
2. **Reducing Swelling**: DMSO's anti-inflammatory effects can dramatically

reduce the swelling around the inflamed tendon, improving mobility and flexibility.

3. **Promoting Healing**: DMSO can enhance tissue repair by increasing blood flow to the affected area, promoting faster recovery from tendon injuries or inflammation.

Bursitis

Bursitis occurs when the small, fluid-filled sacs (bursae) that cushion the joints become inflamed, leading to pain and stiffness. It commonly affects areas like the shoulders, hips, and elbows. DMSO's anti-inflammatory and circulatory benefits are similarly helpful for treating bursitis.

How DMSO Helps with Bursitis:

1. **Reducing Inflammation**: DMSO targets the inflammation in the bursae, reducing swelling and alleviating pain. This can make movement much less painful.

2. **Soothing Pain**: The topical application of DMSO provides immediate relief from the discomfort caused by bursitis, helping individuals regain functionality.

3. **Enhancing Recovery**: By improving circulation and delivering nutrients to the inflamed area, DMSO speeds up the healing process and may reduce the likelihood of recurring flare-ups.

Potential Benefits for Fibromyalgia and Lupus

Fibromyalgia and lupus are both autoimmune disorders that involve widespread inflammation and pain. These conditions are often difficult to manage, requiring ongoing treatment and lifestyle modifications. DMSO offers potential benefits for individuals with these conditions due to its ability to reduce inflammation, ease pain, and enhance the body's natural healing processes.

Fibromyalgia

Fibromyalgia is a chronic condition characterised by widespread pain, tenderness, and fatigue. While the exact cause of fibromyalgia is unknown, it is believed to involve an overactive nervous system and an inflammatory response. DMSO may help to alleviate fibromyalgia symptoms by targeting the inflammation in the muscles and tissues.

How DMSO Helps with Fibromyalgia:

1. **Pain Relief**: DMSO's potent analgesic properties can help manage the widespread muscle and joint pain that people with fibromyalgia experience daily.
2. **Improved Circulation**: Fibromyalgia often leads to poor circulation, which can exacerbate symptoms. DMSO's ability to increase blood flow helps improve circulation, reducing muscle stiffness and tension.

3. **Reducing Fatigue**: By promoting healing and reducing inflammation, DMSO may help to alleviate the fatigue that often accompanies fibromyalgia.

Lupus

Lupus is a systemic autoimmune disorder that can cause inflammation in multiple organs, including the skin, joints, and kidneys. The chronic inflammation associated with lupus often leads to pain, swelling, and tissue damage. DMSO's anti-inflammatory effects and ability to modulate the immune response make it a potential treatment option for lupus patients.

How DMSO Helps with Lupus:

1. **Reducing Inflammation**: DMSO helps reduce the systemic inflammation that can lead to the painful flare-ups experienced by lupus patients. Its ability to penetrate deep tissues allows it to target inflammation in joints, muscles, and organs.

2. **Alleviating Pain**: DMSO's pain-relieving properties can provide relief from the muscle and joint pain associated with lupus, improving quality of life for individuals managing the condition.

3. **Immune System Modulation**: DMSO has the potential to modulate immune system activity, which may help regulate the overactive immune response seen in lupus. However, further research is needed to confirm its role in immune regulation.

Using DMSO for Respiratory Conditions

Respiratory conditions, ranging from asthma and bronchitis to general congestion and inflammation, are common health concerns that impact millions of people around the world. These conditions often result in difficulty breathing, discomfort, and inflammation in the airways, leading to compromised lung function and overall reduced quality of life. Dimethyl Sulfoxide (DMSO) has garnered interest as a potential natural remedy for these types of respiratory ailments. Its powerful anti-inflammatory, analgesic, and mucolytic properties offer promising benefits in alleviating symptoms, reducing inflammation, and promoting overall respiratory health.

DMSO for Asthma and Bronchitis Relief

Asthma and bronchitis are two of the most common respiratory conditions characterised by chronic inflammation of the airways, resulting in difficulty breathing, wheezing, and persistent coughing. Asthma is typically triggered by environmental allergens or irritants, while bronchitis often follows a viral or bacterial infection. Both conditions involve inflammation of the bronchial tubes, which makes it challenging for air to flow freely in and out of the lungs.

DMSO's anti-inflammatory, pain-relieving, and bronchodilator effects make it a promising candidate for managing symptoms of asthma and bronchitis. By reducing the inflammation and relaxing the airways, DMSO can help improve airflow, making breathing easier and more comfortable. Additionally, its analgesic properties can provide relief from the chest tightness and discomfort associated with these respiratory conditions.

DMSO for Asthma Relief

Asthma is a chronic condition in which the airways become inflamed and constricted, making it difficult to breathe. Triggers like pollen, dust, smoke, or cold air can cause asthma attacks, leading to wheezing, coughing, and shortness of breath. DMSO's anti-inflammatory and bronchodilating effects may provide significant relief by addressing both the inflammation and bronchospasms (tightening of the muscles around the airways).

How DMSO Helps with Asthma:

1. **Reducing Inflammation**: One of the core components of asthma is inflammation of the airways. DMSO works to reduce this inflammation, which can help prevent or minimise asthma attacks. By soothing the

irritated tissues and reducing swelling in the bronchial passages, DMSO allows for easier airflow and breathing.

2. **Relaxing the Airways**: DMSO has been shown to possess bronchodilator properties, meaning it helps relax and widen the airways. This can be especially beneficial during an asthma flare-up when the airways constrict, making it difficult to breathe.

3. **Promoting Oxygen Delivery**: DMSO is known to enhance blood circulation, which can improve the delivery of oxygen to the lungs and tissues. This is particularly important for individuals with asthma, as it can support respiratory function and overall well-being.

DMSO for Bronchitis Relief

Bronchitis involves the inflammation of the bronchial tubes, often caused by an infection or exposure to irritants like smoke or pollutants. This inflammation can lead to coughing, mucus production, and difficulty breathing. DMSO's ability to reduce inflammation, relieve pain, and promote mucous clearance makes it an effective option for managing both acute and chronic bronchitis symptoms.

How DMSO Helps with Bronchitis:

1. **Reducing Inflammation**: Bronchitis is marked by inflammation in the bronchi, which can cause the airways to swell and produce excess mucus. DMSO's potent anti-inflammatory properties help to reduce this swelling, making it easier for the individual to breathe and reducing the severity of coughing.
2. **Pain Relief**: DMSO can help alleviate the chest discomfort that often accompanies bronchitis. By reducing inflammation and improving circulation, it helps soothe the muscles and tissues in the chest, providing relief from the soreness caused by coughing and tightness in the chest.
3. **Enhancing Mucus Clearance**: Bronchitis often results in excessive mucus buildup, which can block the airways and make it

even harder to breathe. DMSO's mucolytic properties (ability to break down mucus) can help loosen and expel mucus, improving airflow and reducing congestion.

Using DMSO as a Mucolytic Agent

One of the most useful properties of DMSO in the context of respiratory conditions is its mucolytic effect. Mucolytics are substances that help break down and thin the mucus in the airways, making it easier to clear out and improving respiratory function. For individuals suffering from conditions like bronchitis, chronic obstructive pulmonary disease (COPD), and even the common cold, mucus buildup can be a significant challenge, leading to persistent coughing, chest congestion, and difficulty breathing.

DMSO, when applied topically, has been shown to reduce the thickness of mucus and make it easier to clear out of the lungs. This can be particularly useful for individuals with chronic respiratory conditions that involve persistent mucus production.

How DMSO Acts as a Mucolytic:

1. **Thinning Mucus**: DMSO works by reducing the viscosity (thickness) of mucus in the airways, making it less sticky and easier to expel. This helps clear blocked airways, which can lead to better airflow and less congestion.

2. **Enhancing Mucus Transport**: DMSO may promote the movement of mucus through the airways, facilitating its removal and preventing it from accumulating in the lungs, where it could lead to infections or exacerbate breathing difficulties.

3. **Decreasing Mucus Production**: By reducing inflammation in the airways, DMSO can also help decrease the amount of mucus being produced in the first place,

reducing congestion and making it easier to breathe.

Application Techniques for Respiratory Health

When using DMSO for respiratory conditions, there are several application methods that can be employed, depending on the severity of symptoms and the specific condition being treated. DMSO is typically applied topically, as it is a potent transdermal substance that can easily penetrate the skin and deliver its healing properties to deeper tissues. The most common methods for applying DMSO for respiratory health include direct topical application, inhalation, and as a component of vapour therapies.

Topical Application

For localised relief, DMSO can be applied directly to the chest or throat area. This method is particularly useful for addressing chest tightness, coughing, and inflammation caused by conditions like bronchitis or asthma.

Steps for Topical Application:

1. Clean the area of skin where you plan to apply DMSO to ensure there is no dirt, oils, or lotions that might affect its absorption.
2. Dilute DMSO if necessary (often recommended for concentrations higher than 70%).
3. Gently massage the DMSO into the skin over the chest and upper respiratory areas, where mucus congestion and inflammation are most common.
4. Cover the treated area with a cloth or gauze if you plan to use DMSO for an extended period.

Inhalation or Steam Therapy

Another method of using DMSO for respiratory conditions is through inhalation, often combined with steam therapy. This method can help deliver the therapeutic benefits of DMSO directly to the lungs and airways, where it can have a more immediate effect.

Steps for Inhalation:

1. Add a few drops of DMSO to a bowl of hot, steaming water.
2. Cover your head and the bowl with a towel to trap the steam and DMSO vapours.
3. Breathe deeply through your nose and mouth, allowing the steam to penetrate the lungs and sinuses. Be cautious, as DMSO is very potent and should be used sparingly.

Mucus-Relief Breathing Inhalers

Some advanced preparations of DMSO come in the form of inhalers, which can be used to directly deliver the active ingredients to the lungs. These inhalers are typically used in clinical settings or prescribed by a doctor for more severe respiratory conditions.

DMSO for Digestive Health

Dimethyl Sulfoxide (DMSO) is a versatile compound with a wide range of therapeutic benefits, including its potential to support digestive health. While traditionally used for pain management and inflammation reduction, DMSO's ability to promote healing at the cellular level and improve circulation makes it an increasingly popular option for addressing digestive issues. The benefits of DMSO for conditions like irritable bowel syndrome (IBS), ulcers, gastric inflammation, and even liver support are beginning to gain attention as more individuals seek natural remedies to address their digestive health concerns.

Alleviating Symptoms of Irritable Bowel Syndrome (IBS)

Irritable Bowel Syndrome (IBS) is a common digestive disorder that affects the large intestine, causing symptoms like abdominal pain, bloating, constipation, and diarrhoea. The exact cause of IBS is unknown, but it is thought to involve a combination of factors, including gut sensitivity, inflammation, and dysregulation of the gut-brain axis. Stress, poor diet, and changes in gut motility can also exacerbate symptoms.

DMSO, with its potent anti-inflammatory and analgesic properties, may offer a natural solution for managing IBS symptoms. It is believed to help reduce inflammation in the gut, ease spasms, and support the healing of the intestinal lining. Additionally, DMSO may improve circulation to the digestive organs, promoting more efficient digestion and absorption of nutrients.

How DMSO Helps with IBS:

1. **Reducing Inflammation**: Inflammation in the gut can contribute to the pain and discomfort associated with IBS. DMSO's anti-inflammatory properties work to reduce this inflammation, which can help alleviate abdominal cramping, bloating, and discomfort. By soothing the intestinal lining, DMSO helps restore balance in the digestive system, allowing it to function more effectively.

2. **Muscle Relaxation**: IBS is often characterised by spasms in the colon, which can cause pain, bloating, and altered bowel movements. DMSO has muscle-relaxing properties that can help ease these spasms, leading to fewer cramping episodes and a reduction in the severity of IBS symptoms.

3. **Improving Gut Motility**: DMSO's ability to enhance circulation to the digestive tract may help improve gut motility, which is the movement of food and waste through the intestines. This could be particularly beneficial for individuals with

IBS-related constipation or diarrhoea, as it may promote more regular bowel movements.

4. **Enhancing Healing of the Gut Lining**: DMSO's healing properties extend to the gut lining, which may become damaged due to chronic inflammation. By promoting cellular repair, DMSO could help regenerate the intestinal lining and reduce the permeability that is often associated with IBS (commonly referred to as "leaky gut").

Benefits for Ulcers and Gastric Inflammation

Gastric ulcers are open sores that develop on the lining of the stomach, often caused by an imbalance between stomach acid and protective mucus. They can lead to symptoms such as stomach pain, nausea, and indigestion. Similarly, gastric inflammation (gastritis) involves the irritation of the stomach lining, which can also result in pain, bloating, and discomfort.

DMSO's ability to reduce inflammation and promote cellular healing makes it a potential remedy for ulcers and gastritis. By reducing the inflammation of the stomach lining and improving circulation to the area, DMSO may help soothe symptoms, accelerate healing, and reduce the risk of further ulcer formation.

How DMSO Helps with Ulcers and Gastric Inflammation:

1. **Reducing Gastric Inflammation**: Gastritis and ulcers are both characterised by inflammation of the stomach lining, which can lead to pain, indigestion, and a sense of fullness. DMSO's anti-inflammatory effects help calm this inflammation, providing relief from the discomfort caused by these conditions.

2. **Promoting Healing of the Ulcerated Tissue**: Ulcers are essentially wounds in the stomach lining. DMSO has been shown to promote tissue healing by improving blood flow and stimulating cellular repair processes. By enhancing

circulation to the affected area, DMSO helps deliver nutrients and oxygen to the ulcerated tissue, supporting the regeneration of healthy cells and tissues.

3. **Protecting the Mucosal Barrier**: The stomach has a protective mucus layer that helps shield it from the harsh effects of gastric acid. When this layer is compromised, ulcers can form. DMSO's ability to enhance tissue repair may help strengthen the stomach's protective mucus barrier, reducing the likelihood of ulcer formation or exacerbation.

4. **Reducing Pain and Discomfort**: By reducing inflammation and promoting healing, DMSO can also alleviate the pain associated with gastric ulcers and inflammation. This makes it a valuable option for individuals suffering from chronic stomach pain due to these conditions.

Potential Role in Supporting Liver Function

The liver is one of the most vital organs in the body, responsible for detoxification, digestion, metabolism, and the regulation of blood sugar and cholesterol levels. Given its central role in overall health, maintaining liver function is crucial for optimal well-being. While DMSO is not a cure for liver disease, some studies suggest that it may have beneficial effects on liver function and may support the liver in its detoxifying activities.

DMSO's ability to enhance circulation, reduce inflammation, and support cellular health may help improve liver function by promoting better detoxification and reducing oxidative stress. Additionally, DMSO may assist in the repair of liver tissue and aid in the management of certain liver conditions.

How DMSO Supports Liver Function:

1. **Promoting Detoxification**: The liver plays a crucial role in detoxifying harmful substances in the body. DMSO may support liver function by enhancing

circulation and promoting the flow of blood and nutrients to liver cells, which can help the liver process and eliminate toxins more efficiently.

2. **Reducing Inflammation**: Liver conditions such as fatty liver disease, hepatitis, and cirrhosis are often associated with inflammation of liver tissues. DMSO's anti-inflammatory properties may help reduce this inflammation, alleviating symptoms and promoting the health of liver cells.

3. **Protecting Against Oxidative Stress**: The liver is constantly exposed to oxidative stress, which can damage liver cells and contribute to conditions like fatty liver disease and cirrhosis. DMSO has antioxidant properties, which can help neutralise free radicals and reduce oxidative damage, thereby protecting liver tissue from harm.

4. **Supporting Liver Repair**: If liver cells are damaged, DMSO may aid in the repair and regeneration of liver tissue. By

enhancing circulation and promoting cellular regeneration, DMSO can help the liver recover from damage and function more efficiently.

DMSO for Neurological and Mental Health

Dimethyl sulfoxide (DMSO) is gaining increasing attention for its potential applications in neurological and mental health, offering natural support for brain function, mood regulation, and nerve-related pain. While DMSO is primarily known for its anti-inflammatory and analgesic properties, emerging research suggests it may have significant effects on the central nervous system (CNS) as well. DMSO's ability to cross the blood-brain barrier, reduce inflammation, and support cellular repair makes it a compelling natural treatment for various neurological conditions, including cognitive decline, anxiety, depression, and neuropathy.

Supporting Brain Health and Memory

The brain is a highly complex organ, and maintaining its health is crucial for cognitive function, mental clarity, and overall well-being. As we age, our brain cells can undergo degeneration, leading to conditions like Alzheimer's disease, dementia, and memory impairment. While a variety of treatments and supplements exist for brain health, DMSO offers a promising natural remedy due to its unique ability to cross the blood-brain barrier and promote cellular healing.

How DMSO Supports Brain Health:

1. **Neuroprotective Effects**: One of the most compelling reasons to consider DMSO for brain health is its neuroprotective properties. DMSO has been shown to protect brain cells from oxidative stress,

which can damage the brain and contribute to neurodegenerative diseases. By scavenging free radicals and reducing oxidative damage, DMSO may help slow down the ageing process of the brain and protect against cognitive decline.

2. **Enhancing Blood Flow to the Brain**: DMSO can improve circulation, which may help increase the flow of oxygen and nutrients to the brain. This enhanced blood flow can support brain cell health, promote cognitive function, and help prevent the degeneration of brain tissue. Improved circulation may also aid in the removal of waste products from the brain, contributing to better overall brain health.

3. **Facilitating Cellular Repair and Regeneration**: DMSO's ability to stimulate cellular repair mechanisms may also play a key role in supporting brain health. It encourages the regeneration of healthy brain cells and may help repair damaged tissues, promoting recovery from injuries such as strokes or

concussions. This cellular regeneration is crucial for maintaining mental clarity and memory.

4. **Improving Memory Function**: Memory loss is a common concern as people age or in those suffering from neurodegenerative diseases. DMSO's regenerative effects on brain cells, coupled with its antioxidant properties, may help enhance memory retention and cognitive performance. By supporting the brain's natural healing processes, DMSO may play a role in preventing or reversing memory loss associated with ageing or certain neurological conditions.

Potential Relief for Anxiety and Depression

Anxiety and depression are two of the most common mental health conditions affecting millions of people worldwide. Both are characterised by chemical imbalances in the brain, as well as inflammatory responses.

DMSO's ability to affect both the brain and the body at a cellular level makes it a potential ally in managing these conditions naturally.

How DMSO May Help with Anxiety and Depression:

1. **Regulating Neurotransmitters**: Neurotransmitters are chemicals that transmit signals in the brain, and imbalances in these neurotransmitters (such as serotonin, dopamine, and GABA) are often implicated in anxiety and depression. DMSO has been shown to influence the activity of neurotransmitters in the brain, potentially promoting a more balanced chemical environment that could help reduce feelings of anxiety or sadness.

2. **Reducing Inflammation in the Brain**: Chronic inflammation in the brain, often referred to as neuroinflammation, has been linked to the onset and progression of both anxiety and depression. DMSO's powerful anti-inflammatory properties may help reduce neuroinflammation,

which could lead to improved mood regulation and a reduction in symptoms of both anxiety and depression.

3. **Enhancing Blood Flow to the Brain**: Just as with its neuroprotective effects, DMSO's ability to improve circulation can help with the treatment of anxiety and depression. By increasing the flow of oxygen and nutrients to the brain, DMSO may improve overall brain function, potentially contributing to better emotional stability and reducing feelings of anxiety or depression.

4. **Relaxing the Nervous System**: DMSO's calming effects may help reduce the physical symptoms of anxiety, such as a racing heart or shallow breathing. By relaxing the nervous system and reducing the physical manifestations of stress, DMSO may help people feel more at ease and alleviate the sense of tension associated with anxiety.

5. **Supporting Mood Balance**: The mental health benefits of DMSO may be related

to its ability to support the balance of brain chemistry and its anti-inflammatory properties. As inflammation in the brain decreases and neurotransmitter levels stabilise, individuals may experience an improvement in mood and a reduction in symptoms of depression.

DMSO's Role in Nerve Pain and Neuropathy Management

Nerve pain, also known as neuropathic pain, can result from a variety of conditions, including diabetes, multiple sclerosis, shingles, and injury to the peripheral nerves. This type of pain is often described as burning, tingling, or stabbing, and it can be difficult to treat with conventional pain management methods. DMSO, with its powerful anti-inflammatory and analgesic effects, may offer significant relief to those suffering from nerve-related pain.

How DMSO Helps with Nerve Pain and Neuropathy:

1. **Reducing Nerve Inflammation**: Neuropathy and nerve pain are frequently caused or exacerbated by inflammation of the nerves. DMSO's anti-inflammatory properties make it an effective tool for reducing the swelling and irritation of nerves, leading to a reduction in pain. By targeting the inflammation directly, DMSO can alleviate some of the discomfort associated with conditions like diabetic neuropathy or peripheral neuropathy.

2. **Increasing Blood Flow to Affected Nerves**: Proper circulation is crucial for nerve health and recovery. DMSO helps improve blood flow to the affected areas, which can accelerate healing and reduce pain. Enhanced circulation helps deliver oxygen and nutrients to the damaged nerves, facilitating the repair process and easing discomfort.

3. **Pain Relief Through Nerve Desensitisation**: DMSO has analgesic properties that work by altering the way pain signals are transmitted to the brain. This desensitising effect may help reduce the perception of nerve pain, making it easier for individuals to manage their symptoms. This can be particularly beneficial for conditions like post-herpetic neuralgia (shingles-related nerve pain) or neuropathic pain from spinal injuries.

4. **Promoting Nerve Regeneration**: DMSO's role in promoting cellular regeneration can also aid in the healing of damaged nerves. In conditions like neuropathy, nerve fibres may become damaged or degenerated. By stimulating the regeneration of nerve cells, DMSO could help restore nerve function and reduce the chronic pain associated with nerve damage.

5. **Improving Nerve Communication**: Nerves communicate by transmitting electrical signals to various parts of the

body. DMSO's effects on cellular function may enhance the ability of nerves to transmit these signals more effectively, which can help reduce the severity of nerve pain and improve overall nerve function.

DMSO for Eye and Dental Health

Dimethyl sulfoxide (DMSO) is not only valued for its powerful anti-inflammatory, analgesic, and healing properties in treating various bodily conditions, but it also holds great potential for improving eye and dental health. Its unique ability to penetrate tissues and deliver its therapeutic effects deep within the body makes it an intriguing option for addressing both eye and oral health issues. While DMSO has not yet been widely adopted in mainstream ophthalmology or dentistry, increasing research and anecdotal evidence suggest it can be a valuable tool for improving conditions like glaucoma, cataracts, gum disease, and tooth pain when used correctly and safely.

Potential Use for Glaucoma and Cataracts

Glaucoma and cataracts are two of the most common eye diseases affecting people as they age, and both can significantly impair vision and quality of life. While standard treatments for these conditions are widely available, the use of DMSO in eye health, particularly in alleviating the symptoms or slowing the progression of glaucoma and cataracts, is gaining attention. Although DMSO is not considered a cure for these diseases, it may provide natural relief or be used in conjunction with other treatments.

DMSO and Glaucoma

Glaucoma is a group of eye conditions that lead to damage of the optic nerve, often caused by increased pressure within the eye (intraocular pressure). The condition is typically progressive and can lead to vision loss or blindness if not properly managed. Current treatments primarily focus on lowering intraocular pressure, but they may come with side effects or be ineffective for some patients.

1. **Reducing Inflammation in the Eye**: Chronic inflammation plays a role in the progression of glaucoma. DMSO's powerful anti-inflammatory properties may help reduce inflammation within the eye, potentially relieving pressure on the optic nerve and improving eye health. By reducing inflammation, DMSO can also support the healing process of the delicate tissues in the eye.

2. **Improving Circulation**: DMSO is known to enhance blood flow to the tissues where it is applied. This increased circulation may help optimise the nutrient delivery to the optic nerve and other parts of the eye, supporting overall eye health and potentially slowing the progression of glaucoma.

3. **Anti-oxidant Effects**: DMSO is a potent antioxidant, which means it can help combat oxidative stress, a significant

contributor to nerve damage in glaucoma. By reducing oxidative damage to the optic nerve, DMSO may help preserve vision and protect against further deterioration.

4. **Crossing the Blood-Eye Barrier**: One of the most notable characteristics of DMSO is its ability to cross biological barriers, including the blood-eye barrier. This makes it a promising candidate for targeting eye conditions directly by delivering therapeutic agents to the tissues that need them most.

DMSO and Cataracts

Cataracts occur when the lens of the eye becomes cloudy, leading to blurred vision and, if untreated, potential blindness. Cataract surgery remains the primary treatment, but natural methods, including the use of DMSO, are being explored to slow the progression of cataracts and improve eye health.

1. **Enhancing Cellular Regeneration**: DMSO has been shown to stimulate

cellular repair and regeneration, which could potentially aid in the recovery and maintenance of the lens cells. By promoting healthy cell turnover, DMSO may help prevent or slow the clouding of the lens that causes cataracts.

2. **Anti-oxidant Effects**: Like glaucoma, oxidative stress is one of the factors that contribute to cataract formation. DMSO, being a powerful antioxidant, can help reduce oxidative damage in the lens of the eye, possibly preventing the deterioration that leads to cataracts.

3. **Improving Nutrient Delivery**: DMSO's ability to enhance the delivery of nutrients to tissues may support the health of the eye lens and prevent the accumulation of waste products that could lead to cloudiness. This nutrient support can help maintain the clarity of the lens and improve overall eye function.

Oral Health Benefits: Gum Disease and Tooth Pain

Dental health is an essential component of overall well-being, and DMSO's ability to address various oral health concerns offers a natural, non-invasive alternative to traditional dental treatments. DMSO's anti-inflammatory, analgesic, and healing properties make it effective for treating gum disease, reducing tooth pain, and promoting faster healing in the mouth.

DMSO for Gum Disease

Gum disease (gingivitis and periodontitis) is a common oral condition caused by bacterial infection that leads to inflammation, swelling, bleeding, and sometimes loss of teeth. Traditional treatments for gum disease may include antibiotics, but DMSO offers a natural alternative with a range of benefits for oral health.

1. **Anti-inflammatory Action**: DMSO's potent anti-inflammatory properties can

reduce the swelling and irritation of the gums caused by gum disease. By decreasing inflammation, DMSO can provide relief from the discomfort associated with gum disease and support healthier gum tissue.

2. **Antimicrobial Effects**: DMSO has been shown to have mild antimicrobial properties, which can help combat the bacteria responsible for gum disease. By reducing bacterial growth in the mouth, DMSO can aid in controlling the infection and prevent it from worsening.

3. **Promoting Healing of the Gums**: DMSO helps accelerate tissue repair and regeneration. In cases of gum disease, it can speed up the healing of damaged or infected gum tissues, promoting healthier gums and reducing the risk of tooth loss. The regenerative effects of DMSO help restore tissue integrity, reduce bleeding, and improve the overall health of the gums.

4. **Pain Relief**: The analgesic effects of DMSO can provide relief from the discomfort associated with gum disease, such as tenderness, swelling, and pain. This makes it an effective alternative for those seeking a natural remedy for painful gum conditions.

DMSO for Tooth Pain

Tooth pain can be caused by a variety of factors, including cavities, tooth decay, infection, or trauma. While DMSO is not a substitute for professional dental care, it may offer temporary relief for tooth pain and reduce inflammation around the affected area.

1. **Analgesic Effects**: DMSO is known for its pain relieving properties. It can provide temporary relief from toothaches by desensitising the pain receptors in the affected area. Its analgesic effect is particularly beneficial when combined with other treatments such as warm salt water rinses or herbal remedies.

2. **Reducing Inflammation**: Tooth pain is often caused by inflammation in the gums or tooth pulp. DMSO's anti-inflammatory properties help reduce this swelling, which can alleviate pain and discomfort in the affected area.

3. **Promoting Healing in the Mouth**: If the tooth pain is related to an injury or trauma, DMSO can speed up the healing process. Its regenerative effects support the healing of tissues, reduce swelling, and improve circulation to the affected area, promoting faster recovery.

4. **Temporary Relief for Abscesses**: DMSO may offer temporary relief for tooth abscesses by reducing swelling and providing pain relief. However, it is important to seek professional dental care for abscesses, as they may require more intensive treatment, such as drainage or antibiotics.

Safe Usage for Eyes and Mouth

While DMSO shows promise in improving eye and dental health, it is essential to use it safely, particularly when applying it to sensitive areas like the eyes and mouth. The following guidelines will help ensure that DMSO is used correctly and without causing harm:

Safe Usage for the Eyes

1. **Dilution**: For use in the eyes, DMSO should always be diluted, as its concentrated form can be irritating or harmful. A common dilution is 70% DMSO with 30% sterile saline or water, but it is important to consult a healthcare provider for specific recommendations.

2. **Patch Test**: Before applying DMSO near the eyes, conduct a patch test on another area of skin to ensure there is no allergic reaction or irritation. If any discomfort occurs, discontinue use immediately.

3. **Consultation with an Eye Specialist**: Given the sensitivity of the eye, it is crucial to consult an ophthalmologist or healthcare professional before using

DMSO for eye health. They can advise on the appropriate concentrations and application methods based on the specific condition being treated.

4. **Avoid Contact with Eyes**: DMSO should never be applied directly to the eyes in its undiluted form. If it does come in contact with the eyes, rinse immediately with water or saline.

Safe Usage for the Mouth

1. **Dilution**: When using DMSO in the mouth, it should be diluted properly to avoid irritation. A common ratio for oral use is 50% DMSO to 50% distilled water or saline. Be sure to follow any specific guidelines recommended by a dental professional.

2. **Avoid Swallowing**: DMSO is for topical use, and while it may be beneficial for gum and tooth care, swallowing DMSO is not recommended unless advised by a healthcare professional.

3. **Oral Rinse**: For conditions like gum disease, DMSO can be used as part of an oral rinse. Rinse for a short period (about 30 seconds) and then spit out. This should be done in conjunction with regular dental care, including brushing and flossing.

4. **Consultation with a Dentist**: As with any treatment, it is essential to seek guidance from a dental professional before incorporating DMSO into your oral health regimen, particularly if you have pre-existing dental issues or are undergoing any treatments.

Dosage and Application Protocols

Dimethyl sulfoxide (DMSO) is a powerful and versatile compound with various therapeutic benefits. However, for it to be effective and safe, proper dosage and application protocols must be followed. Since DMSO has the unique ability to penetrate the skin and reach deeper tissues, it is essential to understand how to use it appropriately to avoid unwanted side effects and to maximise its benefits.

Understanding Dosage Guidelines

The appropriate dosage of DMSO depends on several factors, including the form (liquid, gel, or cream), concentration, the specific condition being treated, and the method of application. Since DMSO is highly concentrated and can rapidly absorb into the bloodstream, it is important to start with the lowest effective dose to avoid potential adverse reactions.

1. **Topical Use**:
    - **Concentration**: Topical application of DMSO is the most common method of use, and the concentration typically ranges from 50% to 90%. Lower concentrations (e.g., 50% or 70%) are usually recommended for sensitive skin, while higher concentrations (e.g., 90%) may be used for more targeted or severe conditions.
    - **Application Amount**: When applying DMSO topically, start with a small amount, about a pea-sized amount, and gradually

increase if needed. The product should be massaged into the skin in the affected area.

- o **Frequency**: Generally, DMSO can be applied up to 2-3 times daily, but this may vary depending on the condition being treated and the advice of a healthcare provider.

2. **Oral Use**:

- o **Dosage**: Oral use of DMSO is less common and should be done with caution, ideally under the supervision of a healthcare professional. For oral use, the concentration should typically be diluted to no more than 10% DMSO in water or another vehicle. A typical oral dosage may range from 0.5 to 1 teaspoon (about 2.5 to 5 mL), taken once or twice daily, depending on the severity of the condition.

- o **Timing**: DMSO can be taken on an empty stomach, preferably about 30 minutes before meals to maximise absorption.

- **Safety Considerations**: Oral DMSO is rarely used in mainstream medicine and may cause side effects such as digestive upset, bad taste in the mouth, or skin irritation. Always consult a healthcare provider before using DMSO orally.

3. **Intravenous (IV) Use**:
   - **Clinical Use**: Intravenous administration of DMSO is typically reserved for severe cases and is usually performed in a clinical or hospital setting. The typical IV dosage can vary but generally ranges from 1.5 to 5 mL of DMSO per kilogram of body weight, diluted with saline or another intravenous solution.
   - **Healthcare Supervision**: IV DMSO should always be administered under the supervision of a qualified healthcare provider,

as this method can rapidly introduce the substance into the bloodstream and potentially cause more intense side effects if not monitored correctly.

- ○ **Application Frequency**: In clinical settings, DMSO may be administered one to three times per day, depending on the severity of the condition being treated.

Topical, Oral, and Intravenous Uses

Topical Use

Topical application of DMSO is the most widely used method for home treatment, as it is non-invasive and convenient. The DMSO can be applied directly to the skin or mixed with other substances for enhanced therapeutic effects.

- **Common Uses**: Topical DMSO is primarily used for joint pain, muscle pain, inflammation, skin conditions, and wound healing. It is often used in conditions like arthritis, sprains, strains, tendonitis, and muscle soreness. DMSO is also used for its ability to reduce swelling and bruising.

- **Application Method**: Clean the affected area before application to ensure that the DMSO can penetrate the skin effectively. Apply a thin layer of the DMSO solution directly to the skin and massage gently. Allow the substance to absorb fully, and avoid covering the area with tight clothing or bandages unless recommended by a healthcare provider.

Oral Use

Oral administration of DMSO is more controversial due to the potential for adverse effects and its limited approval for human consumption. Oral DMSO is typically used in specialised settings and for specific conditions, such as urinary tract issues, interstitial cystitis, and other internal inflammation-related problems.

- **Common Uses**: Oral DMSO may be considered in certain medical conditions such as chronic bladder infections, pain management, and inflammatory disorders. It is not commonly prescribed due to limited clinical evidence and the potential for side effects.
- **Application Method**: Oral DMSO should always be diluted, and patients should follow dosage instructions provided by a healthcare provider. It is typically taken with water or another liquid, as the substance can be unpleasant to taste and might cause gastrointestinal discomfort if taken undiluted.

Intravenous Use

Intravenous (IV) administration of DMSO is generally used in hospital settings for acute conditions or severe injuries. It has been studied in clinical trials for its potential in treating conditions such as severe burns, interstitial cystitis, and inflammatory disorders.

- **Common Uses**: IV DMSO may be used to treat severe pain, inflammation, or nerve injuries. It can also be used for its ability to reduce swelling, protect tissues from damage, and promote healing.
- **Application Method**: IV administration should only be performed by a trained medical professional. DMSO is usually diluted with saline or another IV solution and administered over a period of time. Monitoring is crucial due to the rapid absorption of DMSO and its potential side effects, such as headache, dizziness, or changes in blood pressure.

Combining DMSO with Other Treatments

One of the benefits of DMSO is its ability to enhance the absorption and effectiveness of other substances. This property makes DMSO an excellent adjunct to other treatments, as it can increase the penetration of medications, vitamins, or herbal supplements into the body.

1. **With Other Anti-Inflammatories**: DMSO can be combined with other anti-inflammatory treatments, such as corticosteroids or nonsteroidal anti-inflammatory drugs (NSAIDs), to enhance their effects. The combination may provide more effective relief for conditions such as arthritis, muscle pain, and inflammatory conditions.

2. **With Herbal and Natural Remedies**: DMSO is often used to enhance the absorption of herbal extracts, essential oils, or other natural remedies applied topically. For example, combining DMSO with turmeric or arnica gel may provide enhanced anti-inflammatory and pain-relieving benefits for conditions like joint pain or bruising.

3. **With Pain Relievers**: For managing pain, DMSO can be combined with topical pain relievers such as lidocaine or menthol. This combination may provide faster and more potent relief from conditions such as muscle pain or nerve discomfort.

4. **With Antibiotics and Antifungals**: DMSO's ability to penetrate deeply into the skin makes it an effective delivery vehicle for antibiotics, antifungal medications, or antiseptics. When treating infections, combining DMSO with topical antibiotics may help increase the absorption of the medication, allowing it to reach deeper tissues and improve healing times.

5. **With Hydrocortisone and Steroids**: In some cases, DMSO is used alongside corticosteroid creams or gels to enhance the absorption of the steroid, providing quicker relief for inflammation and skin conditions. However, this should only be done under the guidance of a healthcare provider, as the combined effects of steroids and DMSO can be potent.

6. **With Vitamin C or Other Antioxidants**: DMSO can also be used to enhance the effectiveness of antioxidants such as Vitamin C, which is commonly used to promote skin health and reduce oxidative

damage. The combination of these substances may provide additional protection against skin ageing, wounds, or inflammation.

DIY DMSO Blends and Formulas

Dimethyl sulfoxide (DMSO) is a powerful compound known for its ability to penetrate the skin and deliver active ingredients deeply into the body. This makes DMSO an excellent base for creating personalised blends and formulas to address various health concerns, including pain relief, skin healing, inflammation reduction, and more. By combining DMSO with essential oils, natural herbs, and other ingredients, you can create effective and customised treatments at home.

Mixing with Essential Oils and Natural Ingredients

When combining DMSO with other substances, it is essential to use high-quality, pure ingredients. Essential oils, herbal extracts, and other natural remedies can enhance the healing properties of DMSO, and the ability of DMSO to penetrate the skin ensures that these ingredients reach deeper tissues. However, some essential oils may cause skin irritation, so always perform a patch test before applying any blend to larger areas of the body.

1. Essential Oils and Their Therapeutic Properties

- **Peppermint Oil**: Known for its cooling, analgesic, and anti-inflammatory properties, peppermint oil is commonly used to relieve muscle pain, joint discomfort, and headaches. When mixed with DMSO, it can penetrate the skin quickly and provide immediate relief.
- **Lavender Oil**: Lavender oil is highly regarded for its calming effects on both the mind and body. It also has anti-inflammatory, antimicrobial, and

analgesic properties, making it ideal for skin healing and relaxation when combined with DMSO.

- **Eucalyptus Oil**: Eucalyptus oil is frequently used to treat respiratory issues, muscle pain, and joint inflammation. Its combination with DMSO may provide both topical pain relief and support for respiratory health.
- **Tea Tree Oil**: Known for its antibacterial, antifungal, and antiseptic properties, tea tree oil is excellent for treating skin infections, acne, and minor cuts. DMSO enhances its effectiveness by delivering the oil deeper into the skin, speeding up healing.
- **Frankincense Oil**: Frankincense has anti-inflammatory, analgesic, and healing properties, making it perfect for addressing chronic pain, joint issues, and skin conditions. It can also aid in reducing stress and promoting relaxation.

2. Herbal Extracts and Natural Ingredients

- **Arnica Extract**: Arnica is widely used for bruises, sprains, and muscle pain. Its anti-inflammatory and analgesic properties are enhanced when combined with DMSO, providing quick relief for swelling and discomfort.
- **Turmeric Extract**: Turmeric contains curcumin, which has potent anti-inflammatory and antioxidant properties. When combined with DMSO, it can help reduce inflammation, joint pain, and muscle soreness.
- **Aloe Vera**: Aloe vera is well-known for its skin-soothing and healing properties. When combined with DMSO, aloe vera can help to reduce skin irritation, promote healing of burns, cuts, and scrapes, and moisturise dry or damaged skin.
- **CBD Oil**: Cannabidiol (CBD) oil is an emerging remedy for pain relief, inflammation, and anxiety. When mixed with DMSO, it can enhance its pain-relieving effects and promote relaxation.

3. Carrier Oils

Carrier oils are used to dilute essential oils and other potent ingredients, ensuring they are safe for topical use. Some popular carrier oils include:

- **Coconut Oil**: Coconut oil has natural moisturising and antimicrobial properties and can be used to dilute DMSO blends for sensitive skin.
- **Jojoba Oil**: Jojoba oil is known for its ability to balance moisture levels in the skin and can also help dilute DMSO blends, reducing any irritation.

By combining DMSO with one or more of these ingredients, you can create personalised blends that address your specific health concerns, such as pain relief, inflammation reduction, and skin healing.

Creating DMSO Balms and Lotions

Making your own DMSO balms and lotions is a simple yet effective way to harness the power of DMSO for healing and pain relief. The process involves combining DMSO with carrier oils, essential oils, and other natural ingredients to create a topical product that can be applied directly to the skin.

1. Basic DMSO Balm Recipe

A balm is an excellent choice for creating a concentrated formula that can be applied directly to targeted areas of pain or injury. Balms are typically thicker than lotions and provide a more intense, longer-lasting effect.

Ingredients:

- 2 tablespoons DMSO (at a concentration of 70% or 90%)
- 1 tablespoon coconut oil or shea butter (for moisturising)
- 5–10 drops of essential oil (peppermint, lavender, eucalyptus, or frankincense)

- 1 tablespoon beeswax (optional, for thickening)

Instructions:

1. In a double boiler, melt the beeswax and coconut oil (or shea butter) together until fully liquid.
2. Remove from heat and allow to cool for a minute or two.
3. Stir in DMSO carefully, mixing well to combine.
4. Add your essential oils and stir again.
5. Pour the mixture into a small glass jar or tin and allow it to cool and solidify.

How to Use:

- Apply the balm directly to the skin over areas of pain, inflammation, or skin irritation.
- Gently massage it in, allowing the DMSO and essential oils to penetrate the skin.

2. DMSO Lotion Recipe

Lotion is a more fluid option that spreads easily and is absorbed quickly by the skin. This is a great option for covering larger areas or when a lighter, non-greasy texture is preferred.

Ingredients:

- 1/4 cup DMSO (at a concentration of 70%)
- 1/4 cup aloe vera gel (for soothing properties)
- 2 tablespoons carrier oil (jojoba, almond, or olive oil)
- 10–15 drops essential oil (lavender, chamomile, or rosemary)

Instructions:

1. In a clean bowl, combine DMSO and aloe vera gel, stirring well.
2. Add the carrier oil and continue stirring until the mixture is uniform.
3. Drop in your chosen essential oils and mix thoroughly.

4. Transfer the mixture into a small bottle with a pump or squeeze top for easy application.

How to Use:

- Shake the bottle well before use, as natural oils may separate from the gel.
- Apply a small amount to affected areas and massage gently.

Recipes for Pain Relief, Skin Healing, and More

Now that you know the basics of creating DMSO balms and lotions, here are some specific recipes tailored to common health concerns:

1. Pain Relief Blend

This blend is perfect for alleviating joint pain, muscle soreness, and inflammation.

Ingredients:

- 2 tablespoons DMSO (70%)
- 2 tablespoons arnica oil or extract
- 5 drops peppermint essential oil
- 5 drops eucalyptus essential oil

Instructions:

1. Mix DMSO and arnica oil or extract in a small bowl.
2. Add the peppermint and eucalyptus oils and stir thoroughly.
3. Transfer to a small glass container for easy application.

How to Use:

- Apply directly to sore muscles, joints, or areas of inflammation. Massage gently until absorbed.

2. Skin Healing Formula

This soothing recipe is designed for skin conditions, minor burns, cuts, or abrasions.

Ingredients:

- 2 tablespoons DMSO (70%)
- 1 tablespoon aloe vera gel
- 1 teaspoon coconut oil
- 5 drops lavender essential oil
- 5 drops tea tree essential oil

Instructions:

1. In a small bowl, mix the DMSO and aloe vera gel.
2. Add coconut oil and stir until well blended.
3. Add the essential oils and mix well.
4. Store in an airtight jar for use.

How to Use:

- Apply gently to cuts, burns, or other skin irritations. Reapply as needed to encourage healing.

3. Anti-Inflammatory Balm

Ideal for conditions like arthritis or tendonitis, this balm can help reduce inflammation and ease pain.

Ingredients:

- 2 tablespoons DMSO (90%)
- 1 tablespoon turmeric oil or extract
- 5 drops frankincense essential oil
- 5 drops ginger essential oil
- 1 tablespoon shea butter (optional)

Instructions:

1. Melt the shea butter (if using) and mix it with DMSO.
2. Add the turmeric oil or extract, frankincense oil, and ginger oil, and stir well.
3. Pour into a small container and allow to cool.

How to Use:

- Massage the balm into inflamed joints or areas of pain to reduce swelling and promote healing.

DMSO Safety and Precautions

Dimethyl sulfoxide (DMSO) is a potent substance with a range of health benefits, from pain relief and anti-inflammatory effects to promoting wound healing and improving joint mobility. However, its power to penetrate the skin and deliver active ingredients also requires careful handling and awareness of potential risks. To ensure safe and effective use, it is crucial to understand the proper precautions, safe handling methods, and considerations for vulnerable populations.

Safe Handling and Storage Tips

DMSO is a highly effective compound but must be handled with care. Here are the essential safety guidelines to ensure that you use it safely:

1. Storage of DMSO

- **Cool, Dry Place**: Store DMSO in a cool, dry location, away from direct sunlight or heat. High temperatures can degrade the substance and reduce its effectiveness.
- **Sealed Containers**: Always keep DMSO in tightly sealed containers to prevent contamination and evaporation. Because DMSO is hygroscopic (absorbs moisture), exposure to air can lead to degradation and contamination.
- **Avoid Plastic Containers**: DMSO can interact with some types of plastic, breaking them down over time. Store DMSO in glass or high-quality plastic containers designed to handle such substances.
- **Proper Labelling**: Always label the container with the concentration and the date of purchase to ensure you use it

within its shelf life. Over time, DMSO can lose its potency, so it's important to check that it is still effective before use.

2. Handling DMSO

- **Wear Gloves**: When handling DMSO, it is advisable to wear gloves to avoid direct contact with the skin. While DMSO is beneficial for treating pain or skin issues, it can also carry contaminants or substances from your hands into your skin due to its penetrating ability.
- **Avoid Inhalation**: Although DMSO is not highly volatile, avoid inhaling its vapours, especially in poorly ventilated areas. Prolonged exposure to vapours may cause respiratory irritation.
- **Keep Away from Sensitive Areas**: Avoid applying DMSO near the eyes, mucous membranes (such as the mouth, nose, or genitals), or open wounds unless directed by a healthcare professional. Its ability to penetrate the skin means that it could

carry harmful substances into these sensitive areas.

Avoiding Skin Irritation and Other Side Effects

While DMSO has numerous health benefits, it can cause some side effects, especially if used improperly. Most of these side effects are due to overuse, improper dilution, or reactions with other substances. Here are common precautions to minimise irritation and other side effects:

1. Skin Irritation

- **Patch Test**: Before applying DMSO to a larger area of your body, always perform a patch test. Apply a small amount of DMSO to a discreet area (such as the inside of your wrist or elbow) and wait for 24 hours to check for any allergic reactions or skin irritation.
- **Dilution**: If you are concerned about skin sensitivity, dilute DMSO with a carrier oil

(such as coconut oil, jojoba oil, or olive oil) or aloe vera gel. This will help reduce the chances of irritation while still offering therapeutic benefits.

- **Monitor for Redness or Burning Sensation**: Some people may experience a mild burning or tingling sensation upon applying DMSO, especially at higher concentrations. This is generally temporary, but if the sensation persists or causes significant discomfort, rinse the area immediately with cool water and discontinue use.

2. Dry Skin

- DMSO has a drying effect on the skin due to its solvent properties. If applied regularly, it may leave the skin feeling dry or flaky. To counter this, follow up with a moisturising lotion or oil after using DMSO.

3. Headache or Dizziness

- Some individuals report mild headaches or dizziness when using DMSO, especially if they have applied it to large areas of their body or if they are particularly sensitive to the substance. If this occurs, reduce the concentration or frequency of use, or stop using DMSO altogether and consult a healthcare provider.

4. Odour

- DMSO is known for having a distinctive garlic-like odour. This is a harmless, temporary side effect caused by the breakdown of sulphur compounds in DMSO. The smell may persist for a while after application, but it is not usually a cause for concern. If you find the odour unpleasant, try mixing DMSO with essential oils like lavender or eucalyptus to mask the scent.

Guidelines for Sensitive Populations (Children, Elderly, Pregnant Women)

While DMSO can be incredibly beneficial, its use in sensitive populations must be approached with caution. The ability of DMSO to carry substances through the skin means that special care should be taken, especially when using it on children, elderly individuals, or pregnant women.

1. Children

- **Avoid Use in Children Under 2 Years**: DMSO should generally be avoided in children under the age of 2 due to their more delicate skin and the potential for adverse reactions. Consult a paediatrician before using DMSO on children of any age.
- **Use Low Concentrations**: When using DMSO on children, always dilute it well, typically at a concentration of 30-50%. This reduces the risk of skin irritation or

other side effects. Always perform a patch test to check for sensitivities.

- **Monitor Closely**: Children's skin is more absorbent than adults', meaning that DMSO will penetrate deeper and faster. Always observe the child for any signs of discomfort, irritation, or systemic effects (such as drowsiness or dizziness) when using DMSO.

2. Elderly

- **Consult a Healthcare Professional**: Older adults often have more sensitive skin and may be taking other medications or have underlying conditions that affect their response to DMSO. Always consult a healthcare professional before using DMSO, particularly for individuals who are on blood thinners or have a history of skin conditions like eczema or psoriasis.
- **Start with Lower Concentrations**: Older adults may be more prone to skin irritation, so it's best to start with a lower concentration of DMSO, such as 30-50%.

Gradually increase the concentration if necessary, but only with medical guidance.

- **Monitor for Side Effects**: Older individuals may also be at risk for dehydration, which can make their skin more susceptible to the drying effects of DMSO. Ensure that they stay hydrated and use a moisturising follow-up after DMSO application.

3. Pregnant Women

- **Avoid During Pregnancy**: There is limited research on the safety of DMSO during pregnancy, and its ability to carry substances through the skin could potentially pose risks. Due to its high penetration ability, it is generally recommended to avoid using DMSO during pregnancy unless prescribed by a healthcare professional.
- **Consult Your Doctor**: Pregnant women should consult their healthcare provider before using DMSO or any other topical

treatments. If DMSO is deemed necessary, a healthcare provider can guide the safe concentration and proper application techniques.

General Safety Tips

1. **Consult with Your Healthcare Provider**: Always consult with a healthcare provider before starting any new treatments, especially if you are using DMSO for a specific health condition or in combination with other medications. Your doctor will help determine if DMSO is appropriate for your needs and what the best dosage or concentration is.
2. **Use Pure DMSO**: Ensure that the DMSO you use is of high purity and free of contaminants. Impure or diluted DMSO can cause skin irritation or carry harmful impurities into your body.
3. **Avoid Use on Open Wounds**: Although DMSO can aid in wound healing, it

should not be applied directly to large, open wounds or deep cuts, as it can carry bacteria or other harmful agents into the bloodstream.

4. **Hydration**: DMSO has a drying effect on the skin, so ensure you stay hydrated and apply a moisturiser after use to prevent dryness and irritation.

Potential Side Effects and Contraindications

Dimethyl sulfoxide (DMSO) is widely used for its therapeutic properties, from pain management and inflammation reduction to promoting skin healing and improving joint mobility. Despite its benefits, DMSO is not without its potential side effects and contraindications. Understanding these side effects and when to avoid using DMSO is crucial to ensuring its safe and effective use.

Common Side Effects and How to Mitigate Them

While DMSO is generally well-tolerated, some individuals may experience side effects, especially when used improperly or in high concentrations. It is important to recognize these side effects early and take steps to reduce or manage them.

1. Skin Irritation and Sensitivity

- **Symptoms**: Redness, itching, or a burning sensation upon application to the skin are the most common signs of irritation. This reaction may occur if the DMSO is too concentrated or if the skin is sensitive.
- **How to Mitigate**:
  - **Dilute DMSO**: Always dilute DMSO with a carrier oil (like coconut or olive oil) or aloe vera gel to reduce the chances of irritation. A 50% concentration or lower is often a good starting point,

particularly for those with sensitive skin.

- ○ **Patch Test**: Before applying DMSO to a large area, conduct a patch test on a small area of skin (e.g., inside of the elbow or wrist). Wait 24 hours to ensure there are no adverse reactions.
- ○ **Moisturise After Application**: DMSO has a drying effect on the skin, so it's important to apply a hydrating lotion or moisturiser after using it to prevent excessive dryness or flaking.

2. Headache or Dizziness

- **Symptoms**: Some individuals report mild headaches or dizziness after using DMSO, particularly when applied over a large surface area. This may be due to the rapid absorption of the compound or its systemic effects.
- **How to Mitigate**:

- o **Lower Concentration**: If you experience headaches or dizziness, try using a lower concentration of DMSO. Starting with a lower dose allows your body to acclimate to the substance.
- o **Limit Area of Application**: Apply DMSO to smaller areas of the body to reduce the overall absorption rate. This may lessen the likelihood of side effects like headaches.
- o **Stay Hydrated**: DMSO can have a dehydrating effect on the body, so make sure to drink plenty of water before and after use.

3. Garlic-Like Odour

- **Symptoms**: DMSO is notorious for producing a strong, garlic-like odour after application, which can linger for some time.
- **How to Mitigate**:
  - o **Essential Oils**: To mask the odour, mix DMSO with essential oils such

as lavender, peppermint, or eucalyptus. These oils not only help neutralise the smell but also enhance the therapeutic properties of DMSO.

- o **Ventilate the Area**: Ensure proper ventilation when applying DMSO to avoid inhaling the vapour and to reduce the odour buildup.

4. Gastrointestinal Distress

- **Symptoms**: Some people may experience nausea, diarrhoea, or other gastrointestinal issues when DMSO is taken orally or when it is absorbed through the skin and interacts with the digestive system.
- **How to Mitigate**:
  - o **Topical Use**: Avoid oral ingestion unless under the direct guidance of a healthcare professional. Using DMSO topically or as a gel or cream on the skin can help avoid gastrointestinal side effects.

- o **Consult a Doctor**: If gastrointestinal issues arise, stop using DMSO and consult a healthcare provider to determine the cause.

5. Allergic Reactions

- **Symptoms**: Although rare, some individuals may experience allergic reactions, including rash, swelling, or difficulty breathing.
- **How to Mitigate**:
  - o **Stop Use Immediately**: If you experience any signs of an allergic reaction, such as swelling, difficulty breathing, or a rash, stop using DMSO immediately and seek medical attention.
  - o **Consult a Healthcare Provider**: Before using DMSO for the first time, consult with a healthcare provider, especially if you have a history of allergies or sensitivities.

Who Should Avoid DMSO

While DMSO is safe for most people when used appropriately, certain groups should avoid its use altogether or only use it under the guidance of a medical professional. These individuals include:

1. Pregnant Women

- **Risk to Foetus**: The safety of DMSO during pregnancy has not been extensively studied, and there are concerns that DMSO's ability to penetrate the skin and carry substances into the bloodstream could potentially harm the foetus.
- **Recommendation**: Pregnant women should avoid using DMSO unless specifically recommended by a doctor. Always consult with a healthcare provider before using any topical treatments during pregnancy.

2. Children Under the Age of 2

- **Sensitivity**: Children, especially infants, have more sensitive skin and thinner skin barriers, which means DMSO can be absorbed more rapidly and potentially cause harmful effects.
- **Recommendation**: Avoid using DMSO on children under 2 years of age unless specifically prescribed by a healthcare provider. For children older than 2, use only diluted forms and in small quantities, and always under medical supervision.

3. Individuals with Kidney or Liver Disease

- **Potential Strain**: DMSO is metabolised in the liver and kidneys, and its potent effects on the body may put additional strain on already compromised organs.
- **Recommendation**: Individuals with kidney or liver disease should consult a doctor before using DMSO. Healthcare providers may recommend a lower concentration or alternative treatments.

4. People with Allergies to Sulphur Compounds

- **Sulphur Sensitivity**: DMSO contains sulphur, and people with allergies to sulphur or other sulphur-containing compounds may experience allergic reactions when using DMSO.
- **Recommendation**: Avoid DMSO if you have a known sensitivity to sulphur. Always check with your healthcare provider for suitable alternatives.

Drug Interactions and Medical Contraindications

DMSO is known to have the ability to penetrate the skin and bring other substances along with it. As a result, it can potentially interact with other medications, either enhancing their effects or causing unforeseen complications. Below are some of the most notable drug interactions and medical contraindications:

1. Blood Thinners (Anticoagulants)

- **Interaction**: DMSO may enhance the effects of blood thinners such as warfarin, increasing the risk of bleeding. DMSO's ability to carry substances through the skin means that it could increase the absorption of anticoagulant medications applied topically.
- **Recommendation**: People taking blood thinners should consult with their healthcare provider before using DMSO, as it may require adjustment of their medication dosage or careful monitoring.

2. Topical Steroids and Other Topical Medications

- **Interaction**: DMSO can increase the absorption of other topical medications, including steroids or other treatments for skin conditions. This may lead to excessive or unintended systemic absorption of the drug.

- **Recommendation**: If you are using any other topical treatments (e.g., corticosteroids or anti-fungal creams), consult a healthcare provider before using DMSO to avoid excessive absorption of the active ingredients.

3. Diuretics (Water Pills)

- **Interaction**: Diuretics help the body eliminate excess salt and water, and using them with DMSO may alter the effectiveness of the diuretic by enhancing its absorption.
- **Recommendation**: People taking diuretics should use DMSO cautiously and consult with their healthcare provider to ensure there are no complications or changes in drug efficacy.

4. Neurological Medications (e.g., Antidepressants, Anticonvulsants)

- **Interaction**: DMSO may interact with medications that affect the central nervous system (CNS), such as antidepressants, antipsychotics, or anticonvulsants. Since DMSO can increase the absorption of these drugs, it may lead to higher than expected blood levels.

- **Recommendation**: Always consult with a healthcare provider before using DMSO if you are on neurological medications to avoid adverse interactions.

5. Topical Antiseptics and Antibiotics

- **Interaction**: If DMSO is used in combination with topical antiseptics or antibiotics, it may alter their effectiveness or increase the risk of skin irritation.

- **Recommendation**: When using DMSO on wounds or infections, make sure to consult your doctor to determine the best treatment plan and avoid any negative drug interactions.

Combining DMSO with Other Natural Remedies

Dimethyl sulfoxide (DMSO) has gained recognition for its versatile therapeutic properties, but it is often even more effective when combined with other natural remedies. These synergistic effects can amplify the benefits of DMSO and provide more comprehensive support for conditions like pain, inflammation, skin healing, and muscle recovery. In this section, we will explain how DMSO can be combined with other natural substances such as MSM (Methylsulfonylmethane), CBD, and various supplements, as well as its potential benefits when used in conjunction with physical therapy.

Synergistic Effects with MSM (Methylsulfonylmethane)

MSM (Methylsulfonylmethane) is a naturally occurring sulphur compound found in various foods and plants. It is known for its anti-inflammatory, analgesic, and joint-supporting properties. When combined with DMSO, MSM can enhance the therapeutic effects of both substances, making them an effective treatment for joint pain, arthritis, muscle soreness, and other inflammatory conditions.

How DMSO and MSM Work Together

1. **Enhanced Absorption**: DMSO's ability to penetrate the skin and tissues enhances the absorption of other compounds, such as MSM. When MSM is applied topically with DMSO, it can be transported directly

to the targeted area, improving its bioavailability and effectiveness. This is particularly beneficial for treating localised pain and inflammation, as the combination helps MSM reach deep into tissues like cartilage, tendons, and muscles.

2. **Synergistic Anti-Inflammatory Effects**: Both MSM and DMSO possess powerful anti-inflammatory properties. MSM helps reduce the production of pro-inflammatory cytokines, while DMSO reduces swelling and inflammation by increasing blood flow to affected areas. Together, they can provide more significant relief for conditions like arthritis, tendonitis, and bursitis.

3. **Pain Relief**: MSM works as an analgesic by inhibiting the enzymes that break down collagen and other connective tissue proteins, helping to preserve joint health. When combined with DMSO, which has pain-relieving effects, the duo provides a potent combination for managing chronic

pain, especially in conditions like osteoarthritis or after injury.

4. **Joint and Tissue Regeneration**: MSM is known for its role in promoting the production of collagen, a key protein in maintaining the structural integrity of joints, tendons, and skin. DMSO, with its deep penetration ability, facilitates the delivery of MSM to the cells, aiding in tissue regeneration and promoting faster healing of damaged tissues.

How to Combine MSM and DMSO

To use MSM and DMSO together, you can create a topical solution by combining the two in a suitable ratio. A typical starting point is to mix DMSO with MSM powder in a 1:1 ratio (i.e., 50% DMSO and 50% MSM). You can apply this mixture directly to the affected areas of pain or inflammation. It is important to note that the concentration of DMSO should be tailored based on the individual's skin sensitivity and the severity of the condition being treated. Always perform a patch test before applying to larger areas.

Using DMSO with CBD and Other Supplements

Cannabidiol (CBD), derived from the hemp plant, has been widely studied for its therapeutic effects on pain, inflammation, anxiety, and a range of other health issues. The combination of DMSO with CBD has gained attention due to its potential to improve the bioavailability and therapeutic effects of CBD, as well as enhance DMSO's pain-relieving and anti-inflammatory actions.

Synergistic Effects of DMSO and CBD

1. **Increased Bioavailability of CBD**: One of the key benefits of combining DMSO with CBD is the increased bioavailability of CBD. DMSO's ability to enhance the absorption of substances through the skin means that CBD can be delivered more

effectively to the desired area, whether it is pain relief for joints, muscles, or skin conditions. This synergy makes the combination particularly useful for treating localised pain or inflammation.

2. **Pain and Inflammation Management**: CBD has well-documented analgesic and anti-inflammatory effects, particularly for conditions like arthritis, chronic pain, and muscle soreness. DMSO complements these effects by facilitating deeper penetration of CBD into tissues. When combined, the two can offer enhanced relief from both acute and chronic pain, reduce inflammation, and support faster recovery.

3. **Mood and Anxiety Relief**: CBD is also known for its anxiolytic (anxiety-reducing) properties. Using DMSO with CBD may not only help reduce pain but also support mental clarity and emotional well-being. The delivery of CBD to the bloodstream through the skin may help regulate stress hormones and

provide a calming effect, particularly in cases of anxiety and nervous tension.

4. **Support for Skin Health**: CBD is rich in antioxidants and has regenerative properties, making it a popular choice for supporting skin health and healing. DMSO, when applied topically, enhances the penetration of CBD into the skin, helping with conditions such as acne, eczema, psoriasis, and other inflammatory skin conditions.

How to Combine DMSO and CBD

To create a topical solution with DMSO and CBD, you can mix CBD oil or CBD extract with DMSO. It is important to start with a low concentration of CBD and DMSO and gradually increase the dosage based on the desired effect. A typical starting point is a 1:1 ratio of DMSO and CBD oil, but this can be adjusted according to individual needs. Like any other topical treatment, it is recommended to perform a patch test before applying the mixture to larger areas.

Additionally, using oral supplements of CBD (such as CBD capsules) alongside the topical application of DMSO and CBD may provide comprehensive support for both local and systemic effects.

Benefits of Combining DMSO with Physical Therapy

Physical therapy plays a critical role in rehabilitation and recovery from injury or surgery, particularly for musculoskeletal injuries, joint pain, and mobility issues. When combined with DMSO, physical therapy can be enhanced in several ways, leading to improved outcomes for patients.

How DMSO Enhances Physical Therapy

1. **Faster Pain Relief**: DMSO's ability to reduce pain and inflammation can provide immediate relief during physical therapy sessions. By applying DMSO before or after therapy, patients may experience less

discomfort during exercises and stretching, allowing them to engage in therapy with greater intensity and less restriction due to pain.

2. **Enhanced Tissue Healing**: DMSO increases blood flow to affected areas, which can help promote healing and tissue repair. When combined with physical therapy, which often involves the manipulation of muscles, joints, and tissues, DMSO can help accelerate the healing process. This can be particularly beneficial for post-surgical recovery or treating chronic conditions such as tendonitis or arthritis.

3. **Improved Mobility**: DMSO helps reduce stiffness and increases range of motion, which is essential during physical therapy. When used in conjunction with stretching and joint mobilisation techniques, DMSO may help loosen tight muscles, tendons, and ligaments, making physical therapy exercises more effective.

4. **Reduction in Swelling and Inflammation**: Physical therapy can sometimes cause mild swelling or inflammation due to the stress placed on the tissues during exercises. DMSO's anti-inflammatory properties can reduce this swelling and allow patients to continue their therapy sessions with less interruption or discomfort.

How to Combine DMSO and Physical Therapy

For physical therapy, DMSO can be applied topically to the areas of pain or inflammation before and after sessions. A lower concentration of DMSO (around 30-50%) should be used to prevent any irritation or sensitivity. Applying DMSO in conjunction with gentle stretching or massage can help improve flexibility and reduce stiffness. It is important to consult a healthcare provider before using DMSO in this context, especially if the patient is undergoing physical therapy for a serious injury or medical condition.

Additionally, combining DMSO with other supplements, such as MSM, glucosamine, or collagen, may further enhance the benefits of physical therapy by supporting joint health and tissue regeneration.

Case Studies and Real–Life Success Stories

Dimethyl sulfoxide (DMSO) has garnered attention for its diverse therapeutic benefits, but perhaps the most compelling evidence of its power comes from the real-life experiences of those who have used it. From chronic pain relief to accelerated wound healing, DMSO has proven to be a life-changing remedy for many people across different health conditions.

Testimonials from DMSO Users

1. Mary, 52 – Chronic Arthritis Pain Relief

Mary, a 52-year-old woman, had been suffering from rheumatoid arthritis for over 15 years. Her condition had progressed to the point where daily tasks like walking and holding objects had become painful struggles. She had tried various treatments, including NSAIDs, painkillers, and steroid injections, but none had provided lasting relief. Desperate for a solution, she read about DMSO's ability to reduce inflammation and alleviate pain, and decided to give it a try.

Mary began applying a 50% DMSO solution to her affected joints twice daily. Within the first week, she noticed a significant decrease in pain, and after a month, her mobility had drastically improved. "I couldn't believe how quickly I felt relief. My knees and elbows, which had been stiff and swollen for years, started to feel like they could bend again. I've since been able to reduce my pain medication usage, and I feel like I have my life back."

Mary's success story is a testament to DMSO's potential for managing chronic pain, especially in autoimmune conditions like rheumatoid arthritis.

2. John, 36 – Sports Injury Recovery

John, a 36-year-old amateur athlete, injured his shoulder during a game of basketball. He tore a ligament and strained several muscles, which left him unable to lift his arm above his head for weeks. The pain was excruciating, and despite physical therapy, the recovery was slow. After learning about DMSO's properties as a pain reliever and healing agent, he decided to try it in combination with his rehabilitation exercises.

John mixed DMSO with a few drops of peppermint oil for its cooling effect and applied it directly to his injured shoulder every morning and night. After just a few days of use, he noticed that his pain level had significantly decreased. Within two weeks, he regained full range of motion, and his physical therapy sessions became more productive. John credits DMSO for speeding up his recovery and reducing the need for painkillers during the rehabilitation process.

"I was able to get back on the court in less than a month, which was much quicker than I had anticipated. I honestly believe DMSO helped me heal faster," John said.

John's story highlights DMSO's potential for treating soft tissue injuries and accelerating recovery after sports-related trauma.

Documented Medical Cases and Observations

1. Case Study: Treating Severe Burns

A study published in the *Journal of Burn Care & Research* documented a case where DMSO was used to treat a severe burn patient who had suffered third-degree burns on over 40% of their body. The patient had been prescribed standard burn treatments, but healing was slow, and the patient was experiencing significant pain and swelling.

After applying a 70% DMSO solution to the burn areas, the patient's swelling reduced within hours. The DMSO acted as both a pain reliever and an anti-inflammatory agent, providing immediate relief. Within several weeks, the burn wounds healed faster than expected, with a reduction in scarring compared to typical burn recovery cases. The patient reported a significant reduction in pain and a faster rate of skin regeneration.

This case serves as a compelling example of DMSO's potential in enhancing wound healing and providing pain relief in severe burn cases.

2. Case Study: DMSO for Rheumatoid Arthritis

A medical trial conducted in the early 2000s evaluated the use of DMSO as a topical treatment for patients with rheumatoid arthritis. Participants were given either DMSO in combination with a topical anti-inflammatory gel or a placebo. After six weeks of consistent use, those who used DMSO showed a significant reduction in joint swelling, pain, and stiffness compared to the placebo group.

The trial concluded that DMSO, when applied topically, provided a noticeable improvement in the quality of life for rheumatoid arthritis patients. This documented study adds weight to the growing body of evidence supporting DMSO as an effective treatment for joint inflammation and autoimmune-related pain.

How DMSO Changed Lives: Inspiring Accounts

1. Sarah, 27 – Chronic Migraines

Sarah had suffered from debilitating migraines for the past 10 years. Her migraines were so severe that they would leave her incapacitated for hours, sometimes even days, making her life unbearable. Prescription medications would offer minimal relief, and she feared the long-term side effects of constant use. In a search for alternatives, Sarah read about

DMSO's potential to alleviate headaches and migraines due to its anti-inflammatory and analgesic properties.

After starting with a 30% DMSO solution applied to her temples and the back of her neck, Sarah was amazed by the results. "I felt a noticeable reduction in the intensity of my migraines after just a few applications. The pain used to leave me bedridden for days, but now I'm able to function and even go about my normal activities while managing the migraine more effectively."

Sarah's success story is a beacon of hope for others who struggle with chronic migraines, offering an alternative to conventional medications that can often be ineffective or cause unwanted side effects.

2. Mark, 61 – Post-Surgical Recovery

Mark underwent knee replacement surgery due to severe osteoarthritis, which left him with lingering pain and reduced mobility. While the surgery was successful, the recovery process was slower than anticipated. His doctor recommended physical therapy, but Mark also decided to try DMSO as an additional treatment to reduce the inflammation and pain post-surgery.

Mark applied a 50% DMSO solution to the knee daily and noticed a drastic improvement in his recovery. Not only did his swelling and stiffness reduce, but his pain levels decreased significantly, allowing him to perform his physical therapy exercises more effectively. After just six weeks, Mark regained full mobility and returned to his active lifestyle, which included walking long distances and playing golf.

"I credit DMSO for helping me recover much faster than I expected. I still follow my doctor's advice, but DMSO made a noticeable difference," Mark said.

Mark's story demonstrates how DMSO can be an effective adjunct to post-surgical recovery, speeding up healing and reducing pain in the process.

3. Linda, 45 – Skin Healing from Psoriasis

Linda had been living with psoriasis for over 15 years, struggling with flare-ups and irritated, flaky skin that would often become painful and inflamed. After trying various treatments, she found DMSO, which is known for its skin-healing properties. She applied a 40% DMSO solution to her skin daily and combined it with a soothing lotion to help with absorption.

Within a few weeks, Linda noticed a significant reduction in the severity of her flare-ups. The inflammation, redness, and scaly patches began to subside, and her skin became noticeably smoother. "I had tried so many different creams and medications, but nothing worked like DMSO. It's been a game-changer for my skin health," Linda said.

Her success story is an example of how DMSO's deep penetration and anti-inflammatory properties can be beneficial for skin conditions like psoriasis.

DMSO in Veterinary Medicine

Dimethyl sulfoxide (DMSO) is widely known for its therapeutic benefits in human medicine, but its applications in veterinary medicine are just as impressive. DMSO has been used for decades to treat a variety of conditions in animals, from pain and inflammation to injury recovery.

Benefits for Animal Health and Wellness

DMSO's remarkable properties, including its ability to reduce inflammation, alleviate pain, and promote healing, make it an ideal treatment for a range of animal health issues. Here are some of the most notable benefits of DMSO in veterinary care:

1. Anti-Inflammatory and Pain Relief

Just like in humans, DMSO is effective in reducing inflammation and providing pain relief in animals. Its ability to penetrate tissues deeply and rapidly makes it especially useful for conditions involving swollen joints, muscle pain, and soft tissue injuries. For example, DMSO can be used to reduce swelling and provide comfort in animals suffering from arthritis, tendonitis, bursitis, or sprains.

For pets suffering from chronic pain, such as those with hip dysplasia or degenerative joint disease, DMSO can be an excellent adjunct to other pain management therapies. It may also be used for acute injuries, helping to reduce inflammation and promote quicker healing.

2. Wound Healing and Skin Conditions

DMSO is well-regarded for its ability to speed up wound healing, whether in the form of cuts, abrasions, or surgical incisions. It has been shown to help with tissue regeneration and promote faster healing by enhancing circulation and reducing swelling at the site of injury. This makes it an invaluable tool for veterinarians when treating skin injuries in animals.

In addition to external wounds, DMSO can also be beneficial in managing skin conditions such as hot spots, rashes, or infections. By reducing inflammation and promoting cell regeneration, DMSO helps animals recover more quickly from these conditions.

3. Edema and Swelling Reduction

Swelling due to trauma or surgery can be incredibly painful and debilitating for animals. DMSO's ability to reduce swelling makes it particularly effective in managing post-operative edema or swelling caused by injury. It works by dilating blood vessels and improving circulation, which helps to remove excess fluids from the affected area and reduce the pressure on tissues, providing relief to the animal.

4. Treatment of Respiratory Conditions

DMSO's mucolytic properties, which help break down and thin mucus, can be beneficial for animals suffering from respiratory issues like asthma, bronchitis, or other upper respiratory infections. DMSO can help clear mucus from the airways and promote better breathing. When used in conjunction with other treatments, it can support a faster recovery from respiratory illnesses in animals.

Treating Pets: Dosage and Safety Tips

While DMSO can be an effective treatment for animals, it must be used with care to ensure safety and efficacy. The proper dosage, administration methods, and safety guidelines must be followed to avoid potential complications.

1. Dosage Guidelines

The dosage of DMSO for animals varies depending on the type of animal, the condition being treated, and the form of DMSO being used (gel, liquid, or cream). Generally, DMSO should be diluted to prevent any irritation or discomfort for the animal.

For **topical use**, the typical concentration for small animals is a 30-50% DMSO solution. Larger animals, such as horses, may tolerate higher concentrations, typically up to 70%. It's crucial to start with a lower concentration to assess the animal's tolerance. The recommended dose for topical application is generally about 1-2 tablespoons per application area, which can be applied 1-3 times daily depending on the condition being treated.

For **oral administration**, the recommended dosage is usually between 0.1 and 0.5 ml per pound of the animal's body weight. However, oral DMSO should only be given under the supervision of a veterinarian, as improper dosing can lead to potential side effects.

2. Application Tips

- **Clean the Area**: Before applying DMSO to a pet, ensure that the area of treatment is clean and free from dirt, bacteria, or other contaminants.
- **Use Gloves**: Since DMSO is highly penetrating, it's important for pet owners to wear gloves when applying it to their pets, especially when using it for open wounds or cuts. DMSO can carry other substances through the skin, so make sure that only the intended treatment is applied.
- **Monitor for Irritation**: Although rare, some animals may experience skin irritation or sensitivity to DMSO. Always monitor the treated area and discontinue use if any signs of irritation occur.
- **Avoid Eyes and Mucous Membranes**: DMSO should not be applied near sensitive areas like the eyes, nose, or mucous membranes. If DMSO comes into

contact with these areas, rinse thoroughly with water and consult a veterinarian if irritation persists.

3. Safety Precautions

- **Consult a Veterinarian**: Always consult a veterinarian before administering DMSO to a pet, especially for internal use. They can provide guidance on dosage, frequency, and potential interactions with other medications.
- **Store Properly**: DMSO should be stored in a cool, dry place away from sunlight. It's important to keep the medication out of reach of children and pets.
- **Observe for Side Effects**: Although side effects from DMSO are rare, always keep an eye on your pet for any signs of discomfort or adverse reactions, such as increased lethargy, vomiting, or changes in behaviour. If any of these symptoms occur, contact your vet immediately.

DMSO for Horses, Dogs, and Cats

DMSO has shown particular promise in the treatment of various conditions in horses, dogs, and cats, making it a valuable tool in veterinary medicine for these animals.

1. DMSO for Horses

Horses are often subjected to physical strain due to the demands of training, racing, and work. Joint and muscle injuries are common, and DMSO is frequently used as a topical treatment to alleviate pain and inflammation in these animals. For example, DMSO is commonly applied to horses' legs to treat tendon strains, sprains, and soft tissue injuries. It works by reducing swelling and providing pain relief, allowing the horse to recover faster and return to activity.

Additionally, DMSO is used to manage conditions such as laminitis (inflammation of the hoof) and other inflammatory conditions in horses. In these cases, DMSO is typically applied topically to affected areas, either in its pure form or diluted, depending on the severity of the condition.

2. DMSO for Dogs

For dogs, DMSO is most commonly used for its anti-inflammatory properties. Conditions such as arthritis, hip dysplasia, and soft tissue injuries can be managed effectively with DMSO. It can be applied topically to areas affected by pain or swelling, providing immediate relief and helping to reduce the discomfort associated with these conditions.

In some cases, DMSO has been used for acute injuries, such as sprains or muscle strains, to promote faster healing. It may also be used as part of a treatment plan for nerve pain or post-surgical recovery.

3. DMSO for Cats

Cats are more sensitive to certain medications, so the use of DMSO in cats requires careful consideration. However, DMSO can still be an effective treatment for managing inflammation and pain in conditions like arthritis or sprains. It should be used cautiously and in lower concentrations compared to dogs or horses. For cats, DMSO is typically used topically, and the area should be monitored for any signs of irritation.

One common use of DMSO in cats is in the treatment of inflammatory conditions like cystitis (bladder inflammation). By reducing swelling in the urinary tract, DMSO can help alleviate the discomfort associated with this condition.

The Future of DMSO in Medicine

Dimethyl sulfoxide (DMSO) has already made a significant impact in various medical fields, particularly due to its remarkable ability to reduce inflammation, alleviate pain, and enhance the delivery of drugs and other treatments. Despite its long history of use, DMSO continues to evolve in the medical world, with ongoing research uncovering new applications and potential benefits. The future of DMSO in medicine is promising, with exciting developments in areas like cancer therapy, neurological disorders, and other chronic health conditions. This section explores the latest research, emerging applications, and how DMSO is shaping the future of natural medicine.

Latest Research and Emerging Applications

While DMSO has been used for decades as a treatment for various conditions such as arthritis, muscle injuries, and inflammation, recent advancements in medical research are unlocking a broader scope of its potential applications. Researchers are investigating how DMSO might be used in conjunction with cutting-edge therapies to enhance their effectiveness and even revolutionise certain treatments. Some of the most exciting research focuses on DMSO's role in drug delivery systems, as well as its potential use in advanced treatments for diseases like cancer and Alzheimer's.

1. Drug Delivery and Nanomedicine

One of the most promising areas of DMSO research is its use as a carrier or solvent for drug delivery. Because of its ability to penetrate biological membranes and enhance the absorption of other compounds, DMSO is being studied as a potential carrier for a variety of drugs, including those used in chemotherapy, pain management, and chronic diseases.

Recent studies have suggested that DMSO can improve the bioavailability of certain medications, allowing for lower doses and reducing side effects. This is particularly important in treatments that require high doses, such as chemotherapy for cancer. DMSO's ability to facilitate the absorption of drugs across cell membranes may lead to more effective and less invasive drug delivery methods.

Moreover, DMSO is being explored in **nanomedicine**, where it could be used to enhance the delivery of nanoparticles and other therapeutic agents directly to targeted tissues or organs. Nanoparticles are increasingly being used in drug development for their ability to target specific areas of the body with high precision. DMSO could improve the transport of these nanoparticles, making treatments more efficient and reducing the need for invasive procedures.

2. Tissue Regeneration and Healing

Another key area of interest is DMSO's potential for accelerating tissue regeneration. As regenerative medicine advances, DMSO is being investigated for its ability to promote healing and tissue repair, particularly in the context of stem cell therapy. Some researchers are exploring how DMSO can enhance the effects of stem cells by facilitating their growth and integration into damaged tissues. This could have implications for treating injuries, degenerative diseases, and even helping with wound healing and organ regeneration.

In combination with stem cell therapy, DMSO has shown promise in improving the effectiveness of treatment in conditions like heart disease, spinal cord injuries, and joint degeneration. Researchers are also investigating whether DMSO can promote the regeneration of nerves, which could have profound effects on treating conditions like neuropathy or spinal cord injuries.

Potential Developments in Cancer, Alzheimer's, and More

DMSO's future in medicine holds significant promise, especially in the treatment of complex, chronic, and often debilitating conditions like cancer, Alzheimer's disease, and autoimmune disorders. While much of the research is still in early stages, here's a look at how DMSO could shape the future of treatment in these areas.

1. Cancer Treatment and Chemotherapy

Cancer treatment has long been a challenging field, with chemotherapy and radiation therapy offering limited effectiveness and significant side effects. DMSO has the potential to play a transformative role in cancer therapy by improving the delivery of chemotherapy drugs. One of the significant challenges in cancer treatment is ensuring that the drugs reach the tumour cells without harming healthy tissues. DMSO's ability to penetrate cell membranes and facilitate the transport of medications could help chemotherapy drugs reach their targets more effectively.

Some studies are investigating DMSO's use in combination with **liposomal chemotherapy** (which uses lipid-based particles to deliver drugs) to increase the precision and effectiveness of treatment. Research has shown that when combined with certain chemotherapy agents, DMSO may enhance the drugs' efficacy, making them more potent against cancer cells while minimising damage to surrounding tissues.

Additionally, DMSO's ability to reduce inflammation may help counteract some of the side effects of chemotherapy, such as pain and swelling. While DMSO's direct anti-cancer effects are still under investigation, its role as an adjunctive therapy in cancer treatment holds significant potential.

2. Alzheimer's Disease and Neurological Disorders

Alzheimer's disease and other neurodegenerative conditions, such as Parkinson's disease, remain some of the most difficult diseases to treat. There is a growing body of research suggesting that DMSO may have a therapeutic role in these conditions due to its ability to cross the blood-brain barrier, a critical challenge in treating neurological diseases.

Studies have shown that DMSO may help protect brain cells from damage by reducing oxidative stress and inflammation, two key contributors to the progression of Alzheimer's disease. Its neuroprotective properties could also be useful in treating other conditions related to cognitive decline or brain injury. Some research suggests that DMSO could enhance the effectiveness of certain medications used in treating Alzheimer's, potentially making them more effective at slowing disease progression.

Furthermore, DMSO's potential to promote nerve regeneration could have applications in conditions like **multiple sclerosis (MS)**, where nerve damage is a central feature of the disease. While much of this research is still in its early stages, the possibility of DMSO helping repair or protect brain cells offers hope for future treatments.

3. Autoimmune Disorders and Inflammation

Chronic inflammation is a hallmark of many autoimmune disorders, such as **rheumatoid arthritis**, **lupus**, and **Crohn's disease**. DMSO's anti-inflammatory and immunomodulatory properties could help manage these conditions by reducing systemic inflammation and supporting immune system balance. While DMSO is already used to treat inflammation in joint conditions, its future role could extend to managing systemic inflammation in autoimmune diseases.

Emerging studies are examining DMSO's ability to modulate immune responses by enhancing the function of certain immune cells and suppressing inflammatory cytokines. This could lead to new therapeutic strategies for managing autoimmune diseases, which often involve long-term immunosuppressive treatments with significant side effects.

How DMSO is Shaping the Future of Natural Medicine

DMSO's role in modern medicine is evolving from a relatively overlooked substance to a key player in natural and integrative medicine. As healthcare continues to shift toward a more holistic approach, with an emphasis on **natural remedies**, **alternative therapies**, and **minimally invasive treatments**, DMSO stands at the forefront of this change.

1. A Holistic Approach to Healing

Natural medicine has gained significant popularity over the past few decades, as patients and healthcare providers seek alternatives to traditional pharmaceuticals. DMSO fits well within this paradigm due to its natural origins (it is derived from wood pulp) and its versatile therapeutic uses. As research continues to demonstrate its benefits across various conditions, DMSO may become a staple in integrative medicine, particularly in combination with other natural remedies such as herbal treatments, essential oils, and acupuncture.

DMSO's ability to enhance the delivery of other natural compounds is one of the reasons it is gaining traction in integrative medicine. It can be used to carry herbal extracts, vitamins, and other therapeutic agents directly into the body's cells, increasing the effectiveness of these treatments and improving patient outcomes. As the field of natural medicine continues to grow, DMSO's unique properties will likely make it a cornerstone of future therapies.

2. Future of Personalized Medicine

Another exciting prospect for DMSO is its potential role in **personalised medicine**.

Personalised medicine involves tailoring treatments to an individual's specific genetic makeup, lifestyle, and health conditions. DMSO's ability to enhance the absorption and efficacy of drugs or natural compounds could play a key role in making personalised therapies more accessible and effective. By delivering the right combination of treatments at the right doses, DMSO could be a game-changer in the era of personalised healthcare.

Frequently Asked Questions about DMSO

Dimethyl sulfoxide (DMSO) has been used for decades in medical and veterinary settings, yet it still raises many questions among users. While it is known for its therapeutic benefits, the confusion surrounding its application, safety, and effectiveness is common. To help clarify some of the key concerns about DMSO, this section answers some frequently asked questions (FAQs), provides troubleshooting tips, and debunks myths and misunderstandings that often surround the substance.

1. What is DMSO?

Dimethyl sulfoxide (DMSO) is a naturally occurring compound that is primarily known for its ability to reduce inflammation, relieve pain, and enhance the absorption of other drugs and compounds through the skin. It is derived as a byproduct of wood pulp processing and has been used for over 50 years in medical, veterinary, and industrial applications.

In medicine, DMSO is typically applied topically, but it can also be used in intravenous or oral forms, depending on the condition being treated. DMSO's ability to penetrate the skin and its anti-inflammatory and analgesic properties make it particularly useful in managing pain, inflammation, and certain skin conditions.

---

2. How does DMSO work?

DMSO works by reducing inflammation and swelling and by providing relief from pain. It is also known for its **penetration-enhancing**

properties, which means it can carry other substances, including drugs and medications, across biological membranes. This makes DMSO an excellent carrier in drug delivery systems, improving the effectiveness of other treatments when applied topically.

In the body, DMSO reduces the production of inflammatory cytokines and free radicals, two key contributors to pain and swelling. Its antioxidant properties help reduce oxidative stress, while its ability to inhibit certain enzymes involved in the inflammatory process makes it effective for managing chronic inflammatory conditions like arthritis, tendinitis, and bursitis.

---

3. Is DMSO safe to use?

DMSO is generally considered safe when used as directed, but it should be handled with care. Since DMSO has the ability to carry other substances through the skin, anything it comes into contact with can be absorbed into the bloodstream. This is why it's important to ensure that the skin is clean and free of contaminants before applying DMSO.

While DMSO is well-tolerated by most people, some may experience side effects, such as mild skin irritation, a garlic-like odour on the breath, or minor stinging at the application site. In rare cases, more serious side effects like rashes, dizziness, or headaches can occur. Always consult with a healthcare provider before using DMSO, especially for long-term or large-scale applications.

Note: Pregnant women, children, and individuals with compromised immune systems should use DMSO under medical supervision.

---

4. What forms of DMSO are available?

DMSO comes in several forms, including:

- **Liquid**: The most common form, often used in both medical and industrial settings.
- **Gel**: Provides a more controlled application, reducing the risk of excessive absorption.
- **Cream or Lotion**: These forms are typically used for topical application and are often mixed with other therapeutic ingredients.

Each form of DMSO serves different purposes, and the concentration may vary. For example, higher concentrations of DMSO are often used for pain management, while lower concentrations may be used for skin and wound healing. It's important to choose the appropriate form and concentration based on the condition being treated.

---

5. What concentration of DMSO should I use?

DMSO is typically available in concentrations ranging from 10% to 100%. The concentration you choose depends on the condition you're treating:

- **For Pain and Inflammation**: Concentrations between 50% to 70% are commonly used.
- **For Skin Conditions**: Lower concentrations, around 10% to 30%, are often recommended to minimise the risk of irritation.
- **For Severe Conditions**: In some cases, higher concentrations may be used under medical supervision, particularly for deep tissue or joint issues.

Always start with a lower concentration to gauge how your skin reacts and increase it if needed. DMSO should never be used undiluted, especially for sensitive areas, as it can cause irritation.

6. Can I use DMSO with other medications or treatments?

Yes, DMSO can be used in conjunction with other medications, but caution is necessary. Because DMSO enhances the absorption of other substances, it can increase the effectiveness and potency of medications applied at the same time. This can be beneficial when using DMSO to carry topical medications for pain relief, antifungals, or antibiotics.

However, there are potential risks. Some medications may not be suitable to combine with DMSO, as the enhanced absorption could cause side effects or toxicity. Always consult a healthcare provider before combining DMSO with prescription or over-the-counter medications.

---

7. How do I apply DMSO?

When applying DMSO topically, it is essential to follow proper guidelines to ensure its effectiveness and safety:

- **Clean the area**: Wash the skin thoroughly to remove dirt, oils, or lotions that could interfere with absorption.
- **Apply a thin layer**: Apply the DMSO gel, cream, or liquid to the affected area and rub it in gently. Avoid using excessive amounts.
- **Wash hands**: After applying DMSO, wash your hands thoroughly to avoid transferring it to sensitive areas, such as your eyes.
- **Monitor for reactions**: If you're new to DMSO, observe how your skin responds to ensure there is no irritation or unusual reaction.

Note: DMSO should not be used on broken skin or open wounds unless advised by a healthcare provider.

8. What are the side effects of DMSO?

Most side effects of DMSO are mild and temporary. Common side effects include:

- **Skin irritation**: Redness, itching, or a burning sensation may occur, particularly at higher concentrations.
- **Garlic-like odour**: Many people report a distinctive garlic-like smell on their breath or skin after using DMSO. This is normal and not harmful, though it can be unpleasant.
- **Dizziness or headache**: Some individuals may experience dizziness or mild headaches, especially when using DMSO in higher concentrations.

Serious side effects are rare but may include allergic reactions, rashes, or difficulty breathing. If you experience any severe reactions, discontinue use and seek medical advice immediately.

9. Who should avoid DMSO?

While DMSO is generally safe for most people, certain groups should avoid it or use it with caution:

- **Pregnant women**: DMSO should not be used during pregnancy without medical supervision due to its ability to pass through the placenta and potentially affect foetal development.
- **Children**: The safety of DMSO in children has not been fully established. Use only under the guidance of a healthcare provider.
- **People with kidney or liver disease**: DMSO may affect these organs, so it should be avoided or used cautiously in individuals with preexisting kidney or liver conditions.
- **People with skin sensitivities**: If you have sensitive skin, start with a low concentration and monitor for any irritation or adverse reactions.

Always consult with a healthcare provider before using DMSO, particularly if you have underlying health conditions.

---

10. What are some common myths about DMSO?

There are many myths and misconceptions surrounding DMSO, often fueled by its controversial history. Below are a few of the most common misunderstandings:

- **Myth #1: DMSO is a "cure-all"**: While DMSO is highly effective for certain conditions, it is not a universal cure. It is best used as part of a broader treatment plan.
- **Myth #2: DMSO can be used for all types of pain**: While DMSO is effective for pain related to inflammation and joint issues, it may not be appropriate for all types of pain, such as nerve pain.

- **Myth #3: DMSO is completely safe and free of side effects**: While DMSO is generally safe, it can cause mild side effects in some individuals, including skin irritation and a garlic-like odour. It should be used with caution.

---

11. Can DMSO be used for animals?

Yes, DMSO is often used in veterinary medicine, especially for treating inflammation, joint pain, and soft tissue injuries in animals like horses, dogs, and cats. However, the dosage for animals differs from that for humans, and it should be used under the supervision of a veterinarian.

Resources for Further Reading and Suppliers of DMSO

Dimethyl sulfoxide (DMSO) is a powerful and versatile compound that has attracted a wide range of interest in the medical, wellness, and research communities. If you're considering using DMSO or are just curious about its applications, several resources are available to help you learn more, and several suppliers can provide high-quality products. However, it's important to be cautious in your choice of resources and suppliers, as the quality of information and products can vary significantly.

1. Recommended Books, Articles, and Research Papers

There is a wealth of literature on DMSO, ranging from scientific research papers to more practical, user-friendly guides. Here are some resources for both beginners and advanced users:

Books:

- *"DMSO: Nature's Healer"* by Dr. Morton Walker
    - **Pros**: This book offers a thorough exploration of the history, properties, and applications of DMSO. It covers everything from its medical uses to its potential in treating chronic pain, inflammation, and skin conditions.
    - **Cons**: Some readers have criticised the book for being overly optimistic

about DMSO's potential and not adequately discussing the risks.

- *"The DMSO Handbook for Doctors"* by Dr. Stanley W. Jacob
  - **Pros**: Written by one of the leading researchers on DMSO, this book provides comprehensive, scientifically grounded information about its medical uses, treatment protocols, and safety.
  - **Cons**: It may be too technical for casual readers who are just looking for basic information.

Research Papers:

- **National Institutes of Health (NIH) PubMed Database**: The NIH is a trusted source for peer-reviewed studies, where you can find up-to-date research on DMSO's effects on inflammation, pain relief, and other conditions.
  - **Pros**: Provides access to credible, peer-reviewed studies, offering

evidence-based insights into DMSO's therapeutic effects.

- ○ **Cons**: Some studies may be complex, requiring a solid understanding of medical terminology and research methods.

- **Journal of Alternative and Complementary Medicine**: Many studies on alternative medicine, including DMSO, are published here. It's a good resource for exploring DMSO's place in complementary treatments.

  - ○ **Pros**: Features articles from diverse authors and perspectives, which may help you get a broader view of DMSO's medical and alternative uses.

  - ○ **Cons**: Articles can vary in quality, and not all studies are conclusive, so it's essential to critically evaluate the findings.

Online Articles and Blogs:

- Websites like *WebMD* and *Healthline* offer accessible articles on DMSO's health benefits and risks. These sources tend to present well-researched information in a reader-friendly format.
  - **Pros**: They are easy to read and provide a general overview, making them great starting points.
  - **Cons**: They may not go into the depth that more academic papers or books offer, and they sometimes focus more on general health tips than specific scientific findings.

---

2. Where to Buy High-Quality DMSO

When it comes to purchasing DMSO, it's crucial to choose reputable suppliers who sell pure, high-quality products. Poor-quality DMSO or diluted versions may contain impurities that could cause skin irritation or reduce the effectiveness of the compound. Here are some popular places to purchase DMSO:

Online Retailers:

- **Amazon**
  - **Pros**: Offers a wide variety of DMSO products in different forms (liquid, gel, cream) and concentrations. Many sellers offer fast shipping and customer reviews to help guide your purchase.
  - **Cons**: It's important to check the product descriptions and seller ratings carefully. Some DMSO products on Amazon might be diluted or not pure, and the quality can vary from one seller to another.
- **Health food stores and natural product retailers** (e.g., iHerb, Vitacost)
  - **Pros**: These retailers typically offer high-quality, organic DMSO products, often formulated with other natural ingredients. They also provide a wealth of customer reviews to help evaluate products.

- **Cons**: Prices can be higher than purchasing from more specialised suppliers, and shipping costs can add up if you're buying smaller quantities.

Specialty Suppliers:

- **DMSO Company** (dmso.com)
  - **Pros**: Specialises in pure DMSO products, including solutions, gels, and creams. They offer high concentrations and formulations intended for therapeutic use.
  - **Cons**: The website may be difficult to navigate for beginners, and the prices are higher due to the focus on purity and quality. Shipping can also be more expensive.
- **PureFormulas**
  - **Pros**: Known for providing high-quality DMSO products, often sourced from reputable manufacturers. They offer both

> topical and oral versions of DMSO, including gels and creams.
>
> o **Cons**: Their range of DMSO products may be limited, and prices can be a little higher compared to larger, more general retailers.

Local Health Stores or Pharmacies:

- **Pros**: You can purchase DMSO locally, which eliminates waiting for shipping and allows you to physically inspect the product before purchasing. Local stores often have knowledgeable staff who can answer questions.
- **Cons**: Not all health stores carry DMSO, and it may be limited to low concentrations or certain formulations. Prices in local stores can also be higher than buying online.

---

3. Online Communities and Support Groups

If you're looking to connect with others who use DMSO for various health conditions or simply want to learn more about its uses, online communities can be a great resource. Here are some active forums and social media groups where you can engage with others:

Reddit:

- Subreddits like **r/alternativehealth** and **r/NaturalHealing** often feature discussions about DMSO, where users share personal experiences and tips for using DMSO effectively.
  - **Pros**: It's easy to find real-life testimonials and ask questions directly to others who have used DMSO for similar conditions.
  - **Cons**: Some advice can be anecdotal and not always scientifically backed. It's important to cross-check any health-related information you find.

Facebook Groups:

- There are numerous private Facebook groups dedicated to people interested in natural healing, pain relief, and using DMSO. Some of these groups are very active, with members posting about their experiences, asking questions, and sharing research.
    - **Pros**: Easy to join, free to participate in, and members are often supportive, sharing success stories and answering questions.
    - **Cons**: Information can be unverified, and some members may promote products or ideas that are not scientifically sound.

Health and Wellness Forums:

- Websites like **Earth Clinic** and **HealthBoards** host forums where users discuss alternative treatments, including DMSO.
    - **Pros**: Provides a broad variety of experiences and discussions on the safe use of DMSO, along with

treatment recommendations for specific conditions.

- ○ **Cons**: Posts are not always moderated, and there may be conflicting advice. Always take caution when interpreting advice from users with no medical qualifications.

Glossary of Terms

1. **Acetylation**
   The process by which an acetyl group is added to a molecule, often used to modify the behaviour of substances like DMSO for specific therapeutic applications.

2. **Analgesic**
   A substance or drug that relieves pain by acting on the nervous system to reduce the sensation of pain.

3. **Antioxidant**
   A compound that helps neutralise harmful free radicals in the body, thereby preventing cell damage and oxidative stress.

4. **Autoimmune Disorder**
   A condition where the immune system

mistakenly attacks the body's own tissues, leading to inflammation and damage.

5. **Bioavailability**

The proportion of a substance, such as a drug or nutrient, that enters the bloodstream when it is introduced into the body and is made available to its target tissues.

6. **Chronic Pain**

Pain that persists for weeks, months, or even years, typically due to conditions like arthritis, back problems, or neuropathic issues.

7. **Cytotoxicity**

The quality of being toxic to cells, which can lead to cell damage or death, often discussed in relation to the potential effects of substances like DMSO.

8. **Dermal Absorption**

The process by which a substance is absorbed through the skin and into the bloodstream. DMSO is known for its ability to penetrate the skin and carry other substances with it.

9. **Dimethyl Sulfoxide (DMSO)**
A chemical compound derived from wood pulp and sulphur that has a variety of medical, therapeutic, and industrial uses due to its solvent and anti-inflammatory properties.

10. **Dosage**
The specific amount of a substance that should be administered, often expressed in milligrams (mg), grams (g), or millilitres (ml).

11. **Free Radicals**
Unstable molecules that can damage cells, proteins, and DNA by stealing electrons, often leading to diseases and ageing.

12. **Gel Formulation**
A semi-solid form of DMSO that is typically used for topical application. It allows for controlled delivery to the skin and underlying tissues.

13. **Glaucoma**
A group of eye conditions that damage the optic nerve, often associated with high intraocular pressure. DMSO has been

researched for potential benefits in treating certain eye conditions.

14.   **Inflammation**

The body's natural response to injury, infection, or irritation, characterised by redness, heat, swelling, and pain. DMSO is known for its anti-inflammatory effects.

15.   **Mucolytic**

A substance that breaks down mucus, making it easier to expel. DMSO has potential uses in treating conditions like bronchitis and asthma due to its mucolytic properties.

16.   **Neuroprotective**

Substances that help protect nerve cells from damage or degeneration, which could be relevant in conditions like Alzheimer's disease or neuropathy.

17.   **Osteoarthritis**

A degenerative joint disease that involves the breakdown of cartilage in the joints, leading to pain, stiffness, and inflammation. DMSO has been studied as

a potential treatment for osteoarthritis
pain.

18. **Oxidative Stress**
A condition caused by an imbalance
between free radicals and antioxidants in
the body, leading to cell and tissue
damage. DMSO is known for its
antioxidant properties, helping to reduce
oxidative stress.

19. **Pharmacokinetics**
The study of how a drug is absorbed,
distributed, metabolised, and excreted by
the body. DMSO's pharmacokinetics is of
particular interest due to its rapid
absorption and ability to cross biological
barriers.

20. **Purity Level**
The concentration of the active ingredient
in a substance like DMSO, which is often
measured to determine its quality and
safety for use in therapeutic applications.

21. **Rheumatoid Arthritis (RA)**
A chronic autoimmune condition that
causes inflammation and pain in the

joints. DMSO is sometimes used to manage the inflammation and pain associated with RA.

22. **Saturated Solution**

A solution in which the maximum amount of solute has been dissolved in a solvent, such as DMSO mixed with other compounds to create specific formulations.

23. **Solvent**

A substance that dissolves another substance to form a solution. DMSO is a highly effective solvent used in a variety of therapeutic and industrial applications.

24. **Topical Application**

The application of a substance to the surface of the skin for local treatment. DMSO is commonly used in this form to relieve pain and inflammation.

25. **Toxicity**

The degree to which a substance can cause harm to the body. While DMSO is generally considered safe when used appropriately, improper use or contamination can lead to adverse effects.

26. **Transdermal Delivery**

The method by which substances are absorbed through the skin and into the bloodstream. DMSO is known for its ability to facilitate the transdermal delivery of drugs and other compounds.

27. **Tendonitis**

Inflammation or irritation of a tendon, often due to repetitive use or injury. DMSO is sometimes used to reduce the inflammation and pain caused by tendonitis.

28. **Bursitis**

Inflammation of a bursa, a small fluid-filled sac that reduces friction between tissues in the body. DMSO is sometimes used for relief in conditions like bursitis due to its anti-inflammatory effects.

29. **Fibromyalgia**

A condition characterised by widespread muscle pain, fatigue, and tenderness in the body. DMSO's potential to alleviate chronic pain makes it a candidate for managing fibromyalgia symptoms.

30. **Gastritis**

Inflammation of the stomach lining, often caused by infections, excessive alcohol consumption, or stress. DMSO has been explored for its potential to alleviate symptoms of gastric inflammation.

31. **Liver Function**

The ability of the liver to perform essential metabolic processes, including detoxification, protein synthesis, and enzyme production. DMSO has been studied for its potential role in supporting liver health.

32. **Musculoskeletal Disorders**

A group of conditions affecting the muscles, bones, and joints. DMSO is used to treat musculoskeletal conditions by reducing inflammation and pain.

33. **Neuroinflammation**

Inflammation within the brain or nervous system, often implicated in neurological disorders such as Alzheimer's and Parkinson's disease. DMSO has been researched for its neuroprotective and anti-inflammatory properties.

34.   **Phytotherapy**
The use of plant-derived compounds for healing purposes. DMSO is sometimes combined with essential oils and herbal extracts in phytotherapy practices to enhance therapeutic outcomes.

35.   **Polyunsaturated Fatty Acids (PUFAs)**
Essential fats that support cell membrane health and have anti-inflammatory effects. DMSO is often combined with PUFAs in formulations aimed at enhancing skin healing and reducing inflammation.

36.   **Systemic Absorption**
The process by which a substance enters the bloodstream and affects the entire body. DMSO is known for its rapid systemic absorption, making it effective in delivering other substances into the body.

37. **Toxic Shock Syndrome (TSS)**

A potentially life-threatening condition caused by bacterial toxins. DMSO has been studied for its antibacterial and anti-inflammatory effects in the context of managing infections like TSS.

38. **Ulcerative Colitis**

A type of inflammatory bowel disease (IBD) that causes ulcers and inflammation in the colon and rectum. DMSO's potential role in alleviating gastrointestinal symptoms has been explored.

39. **Vasodilation**

The widening of blood vessels, which can reduce blood pressure and improve blood flow. DMSO has been shown to have vasodilatory effects, which may contribute to its therapeutic benefits.

40. **Wound Healing**

The process by which the body repairs damage to the skin or other tissues. DMSO has been found to support wound healing by reducing inflammation and promoting tissue regeneration.

This glossary includes a range of terms that help define the key concepts and processes related to DMSO, from its chemical properties to its applications in health and wellness. Understanding these terms can help you clarify the complex mechanisms through which DMSO works and how it might be used to benefit various conditions.